DETOX JUICING

3-DAY, 7-DAY, AND 14-DAY CLEANSES FOR YOUR HEALTH AND WELL-BEING

MORENA ESCARDÓ
MORENA CUADRA

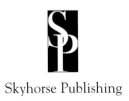

Skyhorse Publishing

Skyhorse Publishing books may be purchased in bulk at special discounts for sales promotion, corporate gifts, fund-raising, or educational purposes. Special editions can also be created to specifications. For details, contact the Special Sales Department, Skyhorse Publishing, 307 West 36th Street, 11th Floor, New York, NY 10018 or info@skyhorsepublishing.com.

Skyhorse® and Skyhorse Publishing® are registered trademarks of Skyhorse Publishing, Inc.®, a Delaware corporation.

www.skyhorsepublishing.com

10 9 8 7 6 5 4 3 2 1

Library of Congress Cataloging-in-Publication Data is on file.

ISBN: 978-1-62914-175-6
E-book ISBN: 978-1-62914-303-3

Printed in China

Notice: This book is intended as a reference volume only, not as a medical manual. It is not intended as a substitute for any medical treatment that may have been prescribed by your doctor. If you suspect that you have a medical problem we urge you to seek competent medical help.

Mention of specific companies, organizations, or authorities in this book does not imply endorsement by the publisher, nor does mention of specific companies, organizations, or authorities imply that they endorse this book. Internet addresses and telephone numbers given in this book were accurate at the time it went to press.

DEDICATION

A mi abue, por nutrir nuestras vidas con su amor y dulzura.

TABLE OF CONTENTS

INTRODUCTION vii
OUR STORY ix

CHAPTER ONE: THE TRUTH
ABOUT TOXINS 1
Toxic Overload 2
The Liver: General of the
   Body's Army 2
The Culture of Overeating 3
The Free Radicals Attack 4

CHAPTER TWO: THE POWER
OF JUICING 6
How Juicing Helps the Body
   Detoxify 7
Hardcore Nutrition 7
Juices vs. Smoothies 8
Does Detox Juicing Have
   Lasting Effects? 9
What Happens after
   a Detox? 10
Ten Reasons to Do a Juice
   Cleanse 11

CHAPTER THREE: DETOX
JUICING 101 12
How Often and for How Long
   Should You Do
   a Cleanse? 13
To Eat or Not to Eat? 14
Is It Safe to Do a Cleanse? 16
Side Effects of Juicing 17
Five Simple Ways to Boost a
   Cleanse 19

CHAPTER FOUR: DIET
RECOMMENDATIONS 20
Diet Dos 20
Diet Don'ts 22
Bitter Is Better 24
Boosting Up Your Juices with
   Superfoods 26

CHAPTER FIVE: O IS FOR
ORGANIC 29
The Poisons in Our Food 29
Where Did the Nutrients Go? ... 30
Organic Sounds Great,
   but Not Everyone Can
   Afford It 31
The Dirty Dozen 33
The Clean Fifteen 33
Cleaning Your Veggies 34

CHAPTER SIX: RECIPES 36
What You Will Need 37
Basics 39
Super Power Greens 51
Not So Green, but Super
   Healthy 95
More Sweet and Fun Options ... 141
Smoothies 169

CHAPTER SEVEN: DETOX
PROGRAMS 184
Three-Day Cleanses 184
Seven-Day Cleanses 186
Fourteen-Day Cleanses 188

RESOURCES 193
RECIPE INDEX 195

INTRODUCTION

The body is the most sophisticated machine we know. We would be fooling ourselves if we thought we could ever entirely understand it, let alone try to outsmart it. So where did the funny idea that we should help something as wise as the body work properly come from?

When we talk about detox diets or "cleanses" this question is the most obvious one to come up. After all, why would anyone need to "clean" their body on the inside when it's supposed to do it on its own?

It's fair to assume that our bodies were designed to breeze us through life without much intervention on our part. But the truth is that, despite the perfect design of each and every one of our cells, at some point, while we were busy being absorbed in our crazy lifestyles, things got a tiny bit complicated.

If you are living the most orderly life, eat only natural foods, use chemical-free cleaners and beauty products, take no medications, drink purified water, buy organic clothes and organic materials for your home, and live somewhere in the middle of the woods, where the air you breathe is still miraculously clean, and where there are no Wi-Fi and no cell phone signals piercing your body 24/7 . . . Congratulations! You are an ace at taking care of your most precious possession: your body. But how realistic is this?

Most people's lives don't have much in common with nature anymore. In the past few decades alone, tens of thousands of new chemicals and contaminants have been introduced into our every day lives. There literally is no place to hide from them anymore, as much as we may try. Our food, the air we breathe, the materials we use, the TV we watch . . . Even the negative feelings we all seem to thrive on these days, like stress, fear, and anger, create toxins in the body and mind.

The unworldly amount of toxins we have to deal with every day put a huge burden on our system. Our body, faithful as ever, tries to keep up. But sooner or later it stays behind with homework. Over time, the body starts storing the toxins it can't get rid of and our detoxifying organs become sluggish from overexertion. The more toxic your lifestyle, the more your body will be ticking like a time bomb, waiting for the last straw to manifest all kinds of discomforts and disease that have been accumulating for a long time in all its secret corners.

The good news is there's a way out of this growing problem. Once you address this issue and start taking adequate measures to help your body protect itself more efficiently from this toxic overload, you can reclaim your health and enjoy the well-being you've always dreamt of (or at least get closer to it).

Just take a look at animals in the wild, and you will get a glimpse at the natural way in which the body heals and replenishes. When animals get sick, they don't go to the vet (unless you take them), and they certainly don't start popping pills, one after the other. What do they do instead? They sleep a lot, and they stop eating solid foods for a day or two. That's all they need to feel shiny and new again.

Healers, doctors, and sages from different cultures throughout history have known this, and that's why bland or liquid diets, or full-blown fasts, are part of many ancient traditions, such as Ayurveda. Giving your body and your digestion an opportunity to rest and repair not only is considered the most effective natural medicine once you're already sick, but also is seen as basic body maintenance that should be practiced regularly to ensure its well-being. Even if you're convinced that your body can deal with the toxic overload of modern life, pampering it by giving it a little rest, and by boosting its immunity with the super nutrition juices provide can't hurt, right?

Believing that chronic health problems and premature aging are a natural part of life that can't be avoided is sad and inaccurate. You are the captain of your ship and with the right information in your hands, and lots of determination, you can take it in whichever direction you see fit. Your extraordinary body is just waiting for you to step up to the plate, and treat it the way it deserves. Once you do, it will respond beautifully. This book will teach you some simple ways in which you can reverse the damage, unleash your inner power, and guide your whole being to lasting health and well-being.

OUR STORY

MORENA E

My first contact with the world of juicing came at such a young age that it now seems like it was destined to become a main pillar in my life. When I was just a kid transitioning into adolescence, my mother would make apple, carrot, and beet juice in the afternoons in her square, bright red juicer. I was a curious kid, so the psychedelic-looking liquid that came out of this strange machine didn't leave me any other choice but to try it.

At the time, I wasn't naturally inclined to eat raw vegetables. I definitely wasn't the one reaching for the salad bowl placed in the middle of the table at lunch. Even though I became a vegetarian when I was four, for skinny ol' me the fun of eating came from carbs, dairy, and especially sugar! Fruits were okay, and so were cooked vegetables depending on what they were accompanied by. Eating crunchy raw veggies, however, was out of the question, as this practice appeared extremely unexciting to my senses. Nobody was more surprised than me when, from one day to the next, I found myself consuming more raw veggies than a rabbit. My love affair with juicing and a healthy lifestyle had begun.

This was the early nineties and juicing was not the big, sexy trend it is today. Certainly not in Peru, where I grew up. One could say my mom was ahead of her time in the wellness area compared to her peers, and I was lucky to be born into her experimental juice-loving nest. The moment she saw my interest in her evening potions, she encouraged me to try them and explained the benefits of drinking them on a regular basis, or even just once in a while. I don't know if I immediately liked them because of their sweetness, because of how intuitively attracted I was to a healthier way of eating, or because I wanted to be like her. Whatever it was, I was hooked.

I've come a long way since then in my juicing adventures. I've spent hundreds of hours in the kitchen assembling juicing machines, washing and cutting up fresh veggies, and throwing them into the mysterious abyss of the juicer, where they disappear with a loud bang and come out at the other end turned into liquid rainbows. I have experimented with all kinds of ingredients, grown my own wheatgrass and herbs, and have a pantry and a fridge bursting with superfoods and wholesome additions for my juices, such as nut spreads, hemp powder, maca, chlorella, and spirulina. In my home we juice every day, and I also do a juice fast for one day every once in a while, to give my body a rest from the daily grind, and, before I quit sugar, from my insatiable sweet tooth.

The positive effects I get from my daily juicing and occasional detoxing are many. My friends always comment on how fresh my skin looks. One of them even jokes that I have a constant "pregnant glow." (But just for the record, I'm not pregnant nor ever have been.) My clothes are the same size they were when I finished high school. Granted, genetics may have a lot to do with that, but something has to be said about the effect my way of eating has had on my slim waist.

Even though I get off track from time to time, I always return to my plant-based vegetarian meals, which include lots and lots of water and fresh juices. The healthier I eat on a regular basis, the more I crave the things that are good for me. One could say eating well is an acquired taste, and juicing even somewhat of an addiction. Once you're giving your body what it needs, it realizes what it was missing out on (real nutrition) and starts crying out loud for it. Once this happens, your relationship with your body will never be the same. Your body will talk to you, and tell you what it needs, at any given time, to thrive. All you need to do is listen. I strongly encourage you to try it.

MORENA C (MY MOTHER)

My mother is not only my creatress and the coauthor of this book, but as I mentioned before, she also introduced me to the fascinating world of juicing, fasting, and detoxing very early on in life. She herself had an early start in taking her health into her own hands, as she went through several periods of spontaneous fasting during her own childhood. These spells lasted up to a week of pure fasting (zero food ingestion and only drinking water), followed by a couple days of juicing. I can only imagine the horror in my grandmother's face as she watched her daughter starve herself to death for no apparent reason.

Nobody taught my mother how to cleanse, or why to do it. It seems like a strong subconscious force of nature came up to the surface about twice a year and told her this was the right thing to do. Pure raw instinct. Do you know what that is? It's that thing most of us have completely lost touch with, especially when we're sitting at the table.

My mother never planned her detox diets, and she never stopped going to school or playing like any other kid while she was at it. Other than the sporadic headache during the first two days, she felt light and exhilarated. Occasionally, thoughts of food came into her mind, but then she realized how clean her body felt without it and the temptation was easily eradicated. Once she started juicing, and eventually went back to eating regular meals, her palate felt more sensitive and she enjoyed the flavors of fruits and vegetables more than ever.

My mom explains her unconventional ways simply: she felt the urge to give her body a rest from food, and when she did she felt better than before. So why not do it? She's now in her mid-fifties and doesn't take a single medication. She also has the body and energy of a twenty-year-old, and not a single wrinkle on her face. So, really, why the hell not?

CHAPTER ONE:
THE TRUTH ABOUT TOXINS

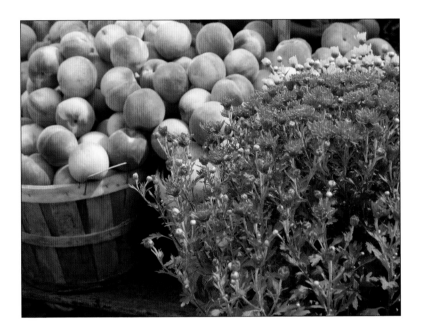

Toxins are all over the place. To completely avoid them is both impractical and impossible. Shampoos, perfumes, plastic water bottles, pesticides in food...Wherever you turn there's a myriad of chemicals waiting to enter your body. The result is that this unnatural way of living throws a far bigger toxic toll on us than our organs were meant to handle.

The problem is not that our detoxifying organs can't do their job well, but that they're given far too much work and they can't completely keep up!

This is the moment when all those itches, aches, and discomforts start appearing, externalizing the fact that toxins have set camp in our bodies.

TOXIC OVERLOAD

Do you always feel like something is wrong in your body yet you can't pinpoint the cause? Do you feel lousy or unbalanced in any way more often than you would like to? If you feel anything but splendid most of the time, your body could be waving its hands high in the air, trying to tell you that it's overwhelmed with your highly toxic lifestyle. (Even if you don't suspect you have a highly toxic lifestyle. By the way, most people do.)

Such symptoms may include:

- Bad digestion
- Chronic fatigue
- Headaches
- Mood swings and depression
- Coated tongue
- Irritable bowel
- Yellow spots on your skin
- Overheating and excessive perspiration
- Acne
- Fat around the waist
- Weak immune system
- Low metabolism
- High cholesterol
- Allergies and rashes
- High blood pressure
- Intolerance to alcohol and medicines
- Heartburn
- Dark circles under your eyes

These are just a few of the problems that an excess of toxins in your body could be causing, and that juicing regularly could start relieving. The list is really much, much longer, as any and all of your symptoms could potentially be caused by too many toxins.

THE LIVER: GENERAL OF THE BODY'S ARMY

The liver is one of your hardest-working organs, second perhaps only to the heart. Its role is to decide what is beneficial and can stay, and also what will cause damage and is inadmissible. It is no coincidence that Chinese medicine describes it as the general of the body's army.

This organ is multitasking for you day in and day out, evaluating everything that enters your bloodstream with an eagle eye, and transforming it into a different biochemical form so that the body can use it as nourishment, get rid of it, or store it as fat in the exact places where you want it the least. This is done by filtering the blood like

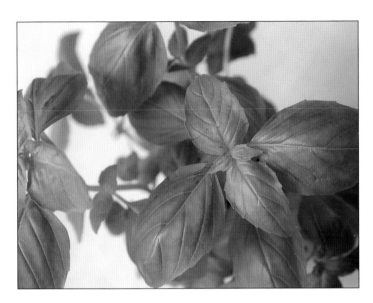

a mega-sophisticated kitchen sieve, singling out the unwanted toxins, and helping them make a discreet exit when you sweat or visit the bathroom.

Despite kicking ass at what it does, there are several factors that can make your liver less efficient at managing its job.

The Culture of Overeating

Can you imagine never giving your car a rest, never taking it to maintenance or changing its parts, and just making it go, go, go? It's pretty obvious that the machine in question would soon start having problems, and eventually burn out. That is if it doesn't explode first! In *The FastDiet*, Dr. Michael Mosley compares the compulsive way we eat, without giving our digestive systems a second's rest, with digging our foot deep in the accelerator pedal of a car all the time. It's strange that most people would never treat their toys and gadgets this way, yet find it acceptable to put that kind of burden on their own bodies. And it's even wilder that they believe their bodies will keep working just fine, without any complaints, despite the unfriendly treatment!

Think about how many times a day you eat a full-on meal, or nibble here and there. Be honest. If you're like most people, the answer is many

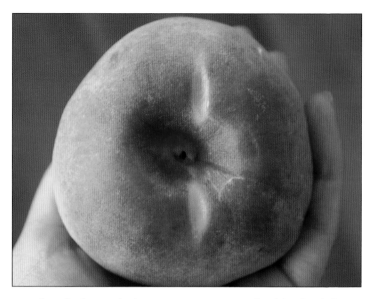

times a day whether you're hungry or not. As a result of this food obsession, our energy is hyper-focused on the sole mission of digesting food.

When we give our digestive systems a rest from solid foods, our energy can be invested in more important endeavors, such as resting, detoxifying, and repairing. Our liver can stop stressing about all the new toxins coming in, and catch up with all the stored ones from past excesses. This is one of the reasons why replacing food with juices during a cleanse is so important. Another reason is that the fruits and vegetables used in large amounts when juicing are packed with antioxidants that help protect the liver from the free radical attack caused by too many toxins and poor nutrition.

The Free Radicals Attack

Free radicals are not just the bad boys most people think they are. They actually assist the liver in getting rid of toxins. Unfortunately, they also attack healthy cells, turning them into free radicals themselves. In turn, these attack new healthy cells and the cascading effect begins. The body, wise as always, has a backup plan for this problem: it produces its own antioxidant enzymes that protect the healthy cells against free radicals. But when there are too many free radicals drifting around, as a result of too many toxins that need to be cleared out of the body, we are eventually unable to maintain this delicate balance.

Detox diets halt the inflow of toxins at least for a while, allowing for a more efficient release of stored toxins. On top of this, the superior nutrition in juicing gives your body the extra antioxidants it needs to balance out all the free radicals produced as a result of our chaotic lifestyles. Are you starting to understand why juices are such detoxifying rock stars?

CHAPTER TWO:
THE POWER OF JUICING

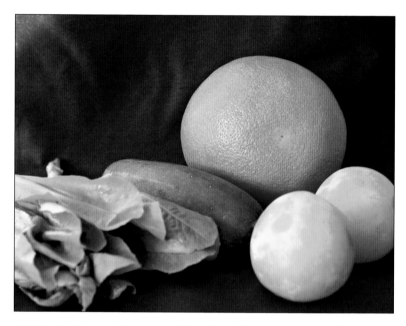

D rinking regular juices is like taking the most potent multivitamins you could ever get your hands on. All the wonderful properties that make fruits and veggies the nutritional powerhouses they are, are trapped in the fiber, and you get only a small fraction of them by chewing your food. When you juice them, on the other hand, you unlock all this nutrition out of the fiber and send it shooting straight into your bloodstream. You could never dream of getting those high doses of nutrients just by eating whole foods unless you were in a veggie-eating contest and ate till you passed out.

Under better conditions the body probably wouldn't need the high levels of nutrition that juicing provides. But we don't live under better conditions, so our bodies could definitely use a hand.

HOW JUICING HELPS THE BODY DETOXIFY

As discussed, when you juice you give your body a break from the daily grind, and your energy can finally stop focusing on never-ending digestion, and start being invested in other repair work. One of the jobs it can now concentrate on more efficiently is ridding itself of stored waste. But there is more.

Hardcore Nutrition

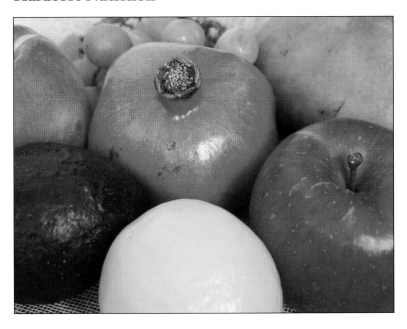

Juicing also helps the body detoxify itself more efficiently by giving it superior nutrition. The high doses of nutrients we get from these drinks are wonderful cleansing agents, as they nourish and stimulate our detoxifying organs, making sure they're healthy and strong. The juices themselves don't clean our bodies. They just help our cleansing organs do a better job at it.

When they get a little bit of help, these organs start flushing stored toxins out of the body in bigger quantities and at a faster pace than when left on their own, or even worse, when being fed a Standard American Diet (very appropriately called SAD). At the same time, getting rid of those toxins helps the body start absorbing nutrients more efficiently, as there is less waste blocking it from doing so. And this makes your organs even healthier and better at detoxifying. This is the replenishing cycle that takes place in your body when you start juicing. Don't you love it?

Even if you keep eating three meals a day and don't go for a full-on cleanse, adding detox juices to your diet will help your body work more efficiently. As an added bonus, they will help you feel fuller and leave less space for unwholesome foods.

Eating processed food without nutrition and full of toxins does the exact opposite. Every time we eat a meal taken out of the Standard American Diet's catalogue, we get little or no nutrition (hence, weaken our organs), and feast on toxins instead. When you do this, you are begging for trouble.

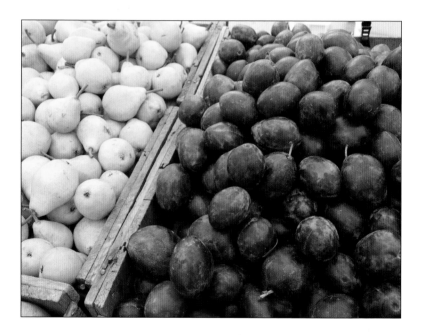

Juices vs. Smoothies

The difference between juices and smoothies is not rocket science. In short, juices are devoid of all the fiber in the fruits and veggies whereas smoothies contain all the fiber. But which one is best?

The answer is they both have pros and cons.

Juices may spike your sugar levels a little, because the fiber is not there to anchor all those natural sugars. However, this can be avoided by drinking greener juices with less sweet fruits and veggies in them. The fact that juices go directly to your bloodstream without any distractions has a super health shot effect on the body. You can actually feel your cells vibrating with vitality and joy when you drink them. Try it, and you'll see what I mean.

Smoothies, on the other hand, take more time to get into your bloodstream, as the fiber still needs to be digested, delaying the process. You also use less amounts of fruits and veggies (hence, less nutrients) in a smoothie, as the bulk of the fiber would make you feel too full if you added more. Of course, this is a pro if fullness is what you're looking for.

All things considered, I prefer to drink juices more often than smoothies, as I get larger amounts of nutrients that way, and they give my body a break from digesting. If you have the time (and the juicer), try to make this your first choice most of the time.

If you have only a blender, however, or if you are always in a rush, smoothies are still a great way of including more fruits and vegetables in your daily routine, and of improving your health by unlocking more nutrients out of the fiber. Just make sure you don't use frozen fruits or veggies too often, as they weaken your digestion (if possible, avoid them completely, or thaw before using), and that you drink them on an empty stomach, and wait at least an hour before you eat something else. Most of the juices in this book can be easily turned into smoothies by adding a little water, green tea, or almond milk to them.

DOES DETOX JUICING HAVE LASTING EFFECTS?

Some nutritionists are against detox diets because they consider them a fad, and a quick fix without lasting effects. I partially agree with this. Detox juicing won't completely change your life if you do it just once and then dive right back into smoking, drinking cocktails every day at happy hour, and having doughnuts for breakfast and pizza for lunch. But if done right, juice cleanses can be a gigantic step toward better health, and greater awareness of your body, how it works, and what you put in it.

To get lasting effects that will be noticeable, you need to accompany your periodic cleanses with a change in diet, and, if possible, a change of lifestyle too. Changing your diet, by the way, is not as hard as you may imagine. Excess eating and cravings are usually the effect of poor nutrition. You may be giving your body large amounts of food every day, but if those foods don't contain what your body needs, it will keep asking for more. Once you start eliminating stored toxins out of your system and your starving cells get a taste of real nourishment, your body will become more efficient at letting you know exactly what it needs.

In fact, one of the great things about juicing is that it is highly addictive. Hooray for that! Once your cells know what they were missing out on, they will never get enough of this royal treatment. Can you imagine how different the world would be if we all had this kind of addiction?

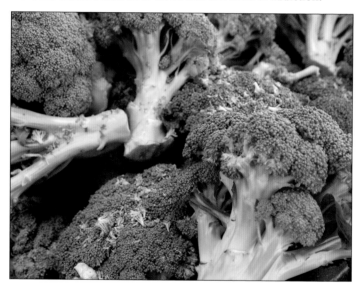

WHAT HAPPENS AFTER A DETOX?

Even if you go back to total food and lifestyle chaos after your cleanse, and only juice and eat healthy once in a blue moon, I do believe that some detoxifying every now and then is by far better than nothing. By bringing your organs back to balance ever so slightly, your body will carry less of a toxic burden for a while, be more efficient at absorbing nutrients, and start working more efficiently than if you never gave it proper maintenance.

But of course, we encourage you to keep drinking these nutrient-rich juices on a regular basis, and to make wholesome food choices for the rest of your life. Doing this will be totally worth your effort.

TEN REASONS TO DO A JUICE CLEANSE

1. You have been eating the Standard American Diet for far too long!
2. You want to know what your body really wants.
3. Your digestive system needs a much-needed vacation from all that overeating.
4. You want to look younger for longer, and to feel it too.
5. It's spring, and you feel the urge to do an internal house cleanse.
6. You want to get rid of your compulsive cravings, and get new, healthier ones in their place.
7. You want to feel amazing for the first time in a very long time, and get rid of annoying physical, mental, and emotional symptoms.
8. You want your clothes to fit better.
9. You want to navigate more smoothly through the physical and emotional toxins in your daily life.
10. You're feeling adventurous and want to try new fruits and veggies every day.

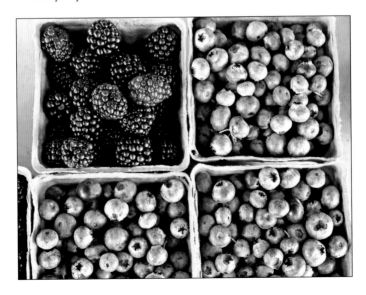

CHAPTER THREE:
DETOX JUICING 101

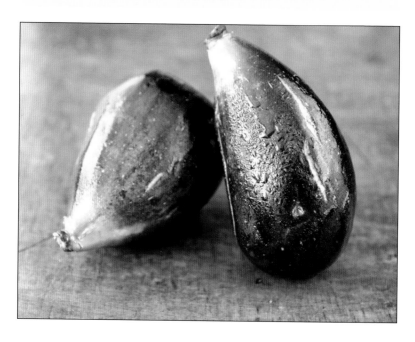

There are many different opinions as to what the best way of doing a juice cleanse is. Some people go on for several weeks drinking only water or only juice, and avoiding all solid foods. And there are those who do both juices and food at the same time.

Then there is the question of time. I have friends who have gone up to three weeks just juicing. They say they stopped feeling hungry by the third day, and had more energy and mental clarity than ever before. Most people, however, prefer doing this for shorter periods of time.

Our approach tends to be of the gentler kind, and we run away from anything radical. When it comes to juicing, we truly believe that the most important thing is that you actually do it! Cleansing in a way that will leave you starved and grumpy, and will be a huge (too huge) test on your willpower, won't do. What's the point of choosing the most life-changing diet if you'll cheat or quit by the second day? We want you to succeed, and to enjoy the ride while you're at it.

HOW OFTEN AND FOR HOW LONG SHOULD YOU DO A CLEANSE?

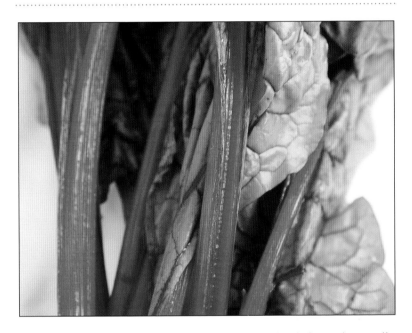

I personally like adding one daily juice to my regular daily meals. Usually, I take this as a snack, or a pre-breakfast or pre-dinner appetizer. If I'm too full from overeating the previous day, or feel a bit undigested, I'll replace dinner or breakfast with a juice, as well.

I also like doing one-day juice fasts every now and then, particularly when the seasons change, or during a new moon. When I do this, I only drink juices and eat no other food. On that day, I have at least three or four juices. I have no problem maintaining these one-day cleanses, as they go quickly enough and I know I can eat whatever I want the following day. I have a very fast metabolism, and feel too weak, and get cold extremities and strong headaches if I fast for longer than that, or if I do it too often. Everybody is different, so you should try different approaches and see what works best for you.

If, after trying, you find that a three-day program works wonders for you, it could be a good idea to do it once a month, or once every change of season, depending on your lifestyle and the state of your health. Seven- or fourteen-day programs can be practiced once or twice a year for optimal results.

Spring is an ideal time to do a cleanse. It is no coincidence that we feel moved to do a spring cleaning of our homes every year. The liver is more active during this season, and cleaning our surroundings is just an outward expression of what's going on at this time of year inside our bodies. So go ahead and cleanse away when you see the first flowers blooming in your garden or hear the first birds chirping.

TO EAT OR NOT TO EAT?

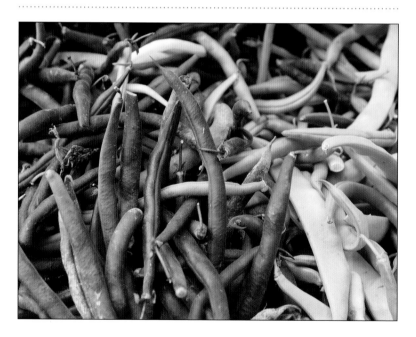

We've separated this book into three-, seven-, and fourteen-day programs. None of them are complete juice fasts, because we want to ease you into juicing, and then let this adventure take its own course in each of your lives. It's better if you start this way, see how you feel, and start experimenting on your own. Try to always stay on the safe side, and if you don't feel well, stop, increase the amount of food, or decrease the amount of juices. Every body is unique, and you should honor your particular constitution.

If you're more of a free spirit and want to create your own detox programs using our recipes, follow these guidelines to have a pleasant detox experience:

- For three-day programs, replace breakfast and dinner with a juice, and have two juice snacks during the day as well. Eat a regular lunch.
- For seven-day programs, we recommend you replace breakfast and dinner with a juice on the first, fourth, and seventh day, and have a big, healthy lunch. Have two juice snacks throughout the day, when you feel hungry. During the other days replace dinner with a juice (choose one of the greener kinds) and have a healthy breakfast and lunch. Again, don't forget to snack on green juices if you get hungry.
- For a fourteen-day detox, we advise that you replace two meals with a juice on the first day, one meal with a juice on the second day, and eat your regular three meals on the third day. However, you should snack on one or two green juices, as always, even on the day when you eat three regular meals. Repeat this process several times, until you complete the fourteen days.

As you can see, in all the programs we encourage you to have one or two juices as snacks between meals if you feel hungry. If you do this, pick the ones with less fruit and more veggies in general. These can be found in the Super Power Greens recipe section.

Try to use this time to start listening to your body closer, and realize when you're actually hungry, as opposed to thirsty, anxious, or bored. Why do you want to eat a particular thing at a certain time? What feelings triggered that craving? What are you trying to avoid, or what space are you trying to fill with that food?

Cleansing is a great opportunity to reconnect with your inner guide, and perhaps dig deeper into your relationship with food, with your body, and with your emotions. If done with awareness, cleanses can impact your life at deeper levels than you would expect.

IS IT SAFE TO DO A CLEANSE?

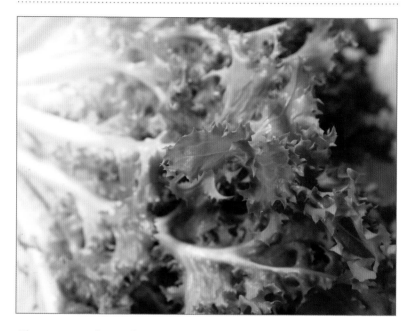

Cleansing is a fun and natural way of pressing the reset button on your body's healing mechanisms. Wise men and women all around the world have been practicing fasting (both with and without juicing) for centuries as a regular way to bring balance back to their bodies, minds, and even souls.

We recommend juicing as a way to enhance your life and health. However, we are not medical practitioners, and talk only from our own lifelong experience with juicing.

As with any other lifestyle and dietary changes, you should consult a physician before starting a detox program, especially if:

- ♦ You have any serious or chronic health concerns.
- ♦ You have an eating disorder.
- ♦ You are taking medications.
- ♦ You are pregnant, trying to get pregnant, or nursing.
- ♦ You feel there is any other reason that may put you at risk. Use common sense to evaluate this.

Even if you're healthy, we don't recommend you follow these programs for longer than fourteen days, unless you are under strict supervision from a doctor. You may, however, keep adding a juice or two to your daily routine after you finish a cleanse, or even replace a meal with one or two juices every now and then if you feel your body needs it. If you're about to have a naughty snack between meals, you can't go wrong by replacing it with a juice.

SIDE EFFECTS OF JUICING

When you go through a cleanse you release toxins stored in your colon, liver, lungs, bladder, sinuses, skin, kidneys, and fatty tissue. The more toxins you've accumulated throughout the years by a lousy diet and a sloppy

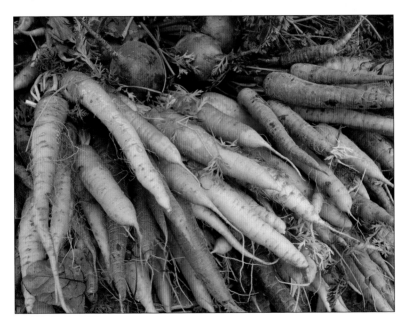

lifestyle, the more you will have to release. This may cause a few unpleasant symptoms that you would probably be happier without. Any discomfort caused by toxicity, such as bloating, phlegm, or acne, may become stronger at first, before it starts getting better.

Experiencing this toxic hump is natural, as the stored waste needs to be released back into your bloodstream before it can exit your body. At the end of the day this downside is nothing compared to the many upsides you will get from sweeping those little buggers out of your body once and for all. Just be patient and you will soon start seeing the light at the end of the tunnel.

> If symptoms arrive, drink lots of water to flush them out of your system quickly. If they are too strong or persist, consider stopping the cleanse and trying a milder version of it in the future.

It may also be the case that you experience no negative symptoms whatsoever, so don't take this potential scenario too seriously. We just feel that for the sake of honesty, it's better to warn you that this may not be a complete walk in the park for everyone.

To avoid a tough ride, make sure you begin slowly, especially if you don't have the most "kosher" of diets. Start getting acquainted with a higher daily dose of fruits and veggies little by little. Ambushing your body with a triple dose of the strongest detoxifying juices, such as the

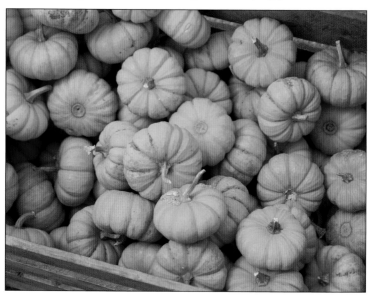

Beet-er Dandelion on the very first day of your cleanse would be a recipe for disaster. Instead, be slow but sure like the turtle, and build your detox practice one juice at a time.

Five Simple Ways to Boost a Cleanse

- Dry scrub your skin first thing in the morning. Our skin is the largest organ of our bodies, and every day toxins are released through its pores. If they are blocked, toxins are reabsorbed and go back into your bloodstream. By scrubbing regularly, you're easing their way out of your system and guaranteeing better-looking skin at the same time. If you leave the scrub in a visible place of the bathroom it will be easier for you to remember, and will become a regular habit just like brushing your teeth.
- Exercise. Moving your body gets those stored toxins moving too, and sweating gets them out. It's as simple as that.
- Clean your tongue when you wake up. Those funny-looking tongue cleaners are much more important than you might think. Most of our body's detoxification happens during sleep, and the white coating on the tongue that most people wake up to is actually a fresh layer of toxins that the body released during the night. If you don't clean it out, you will swallow it back.
- Get a massage. Do you even need persuasion for this one? Digging deep into your tissues and moving them manually also moves what's stuck to them (toxins!). So indulge in this healthy pleasure as often as you want, and drink tons of water when it's finished to help flush them out.
- Go to sleep early. This one is tricky for night owls and party animals, but at least during your cleanse, try to go to sleep at around ten at night (if you're already asleep at ten, even better!). Your liver is the most active at this time, so if you're resting, all your energy can go into its important repair work.

CHAPTER FOUR:
DIET RECOMMENDATIONS

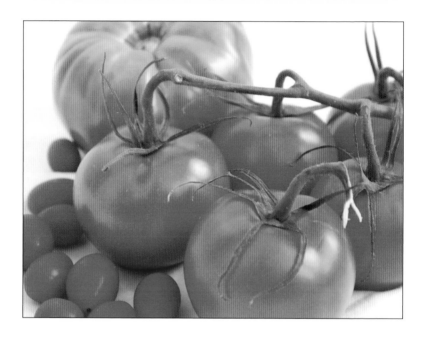

There are some diet tips that should guide you during a cleanse. Whether you choose to do a three-, seven-, or fourteen-day detox program, you should opt for certain foods, and avoid others. Following these guidelines will ensure that you're giving your body what it needs to recharge, and that you're staying away from any offenders.

DIET DOS

- Eat whole grains, except wheat. If they're refined (i.e., white, and with no real nutrients nor fiber left in them), stay away.
- Consume fresh fruits and vegetables freely, and remember that organic is always best.

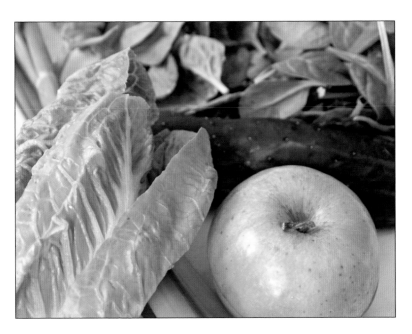

- Raw nuts and seeds are great energy boosters. Soak them overnight and peel them to make them more digestible. Avoid cashews and peanuts during a cleanse, because they're more prone to growing mold.
- Legumes are a great source of fiber, energy, and nutrients. It's even better if they're sprouted, to avoid bloating. If you can't find them sprouted, make sure you soak them overnight before cooking. Avoid canned legumes if you can.
- Fermented foods preserve nutrients and make some ingredients more digestible. They are also full of beneficial bacteria that will boost your immune system and improve your digestion and elimination.
- Spices and herbs add variety to your meals, and variety is the spice of life! Just because you want to be healthier doesn't mean you have to eat a bland diet. Spices and herbs are delicious and packed with healing properties that your body could benefit from.
- Salt is rich in essential minerals, so don't be so scared of it. Just avoid processed table salt because it's devoid of minerals and has undesired additives. Himalayan and Peruvian pink salts are pure and nutritious, as are good-quality sea salts. However, don't overdo it. Give your taste buds a rest from excessive amounts of salt, and discover what food really tastes like.

- Oils are essential to your well-being, but you need to be picky about them. Favor organic cold-pressed extra-virgin olive oil, flaxseed oil, hempseed oil, sesame oil, and coconut oil. Avoid margarine and, by all means, shortening (this is not food!), and heavily processed oils such as corn and canola.
- Herbal teas will keep you satiated, improve digestion, and relax your mind. Make sure you get organic herbal teas, because even these can be covered in pesticides.
- Our body is mostly water, and we need to keep it alive, don't we? During a cleanse you will need it in abundance, to flush all the toxins that the juices will help you release. Avoid water that comes in toxic plastic bottles. Better to drink filtered tap water if those are your two options.

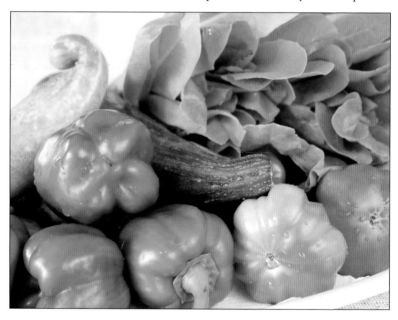

DIET DON'TS

- Alcohol is an obvious no-no during a cleanse. Consuming it while you're trying to enhance your liver function at the same time would be like trying to bake a cake in the freezer.
- Avoid any foods you're allergic to. If you want to go all the way, get an allergy test so you know what to avoid.

- GMOs sound like creatures from outer space, and that's pretty much what they are. Any food that has been genetically modified is not the way nature intended it to be, and may not nourish or help your body heal the way food is supposed to. In addition, GMOs usually come chaperoned by dangerous pesticides and other chemicals.
- Soy and corn sold around the world tend to be genetically modified (read bullet point above). They also are strong allergens. Soy is not properly digested by the body unless it's eaten in its fermented forms (miso and tempeh), so avoid it during a cleanse, and if you're not allergic to it, eat it only if it's organic the rest of the time.
- Gluten is a substance found in wheat that gives that addictive chewy texture to all the products that contain it. Too bad that an increasingly high number of people around the globe are becoming aware that they suffer from gluten intolerance or allergies. The best way to find out if you're one of them is to stop cold turkey for a few weeks, and see how you feel without it. Do not consume it during a detox diet.
- Added sugars should be avoided at all costs during a detox diet and, if absolutely necessary, eaten only in moderation the rest of the time (I know, this is a hard one). Refined sugar is the culprit of many chronic diseases. It's highly toxic, creates inflammation in the body, and I won't even try to list all the other ways in which it's bad for you, because I would never finish. Just. Say. No. If you can't live without it, raw local honey, maple syrup, yacon syrup, lucuma powder, and some brands of stevia are good alternatives. Remember, moderation is key here.
- Artificial sweeteners are toxic for your nervous system and your brain. Get all the sugar you need during a detox from your favorite fruits.
- Meat and dairy should completely be avoided during a cleanse. Here's the most obvious reason why: unless you are consuming meat or dairy from organic, grass-fed animals, you are also eating all the hormones and antibiotics these animals are attacked with in the farms. On top of this, you are indirectly eating all the GMO, toxic food they are fed. Also, meat is hard to digest, so the whole point of giving your body a rest during a juice detox would become compromised. Most people can't digest lactose, and consuming it

creates mucus and inflammation in the body. Hopefully, this is enough to convince you. You will be better off without them during a cleanse, and by decreasing their consumption the rest of the time.

- Caffeine clogs up your liver, dehydrates you, and puts your nervous system in alert mode. This keeps you awake when you're sleepy and need to go to work, but it also interferes with a good night's sleep (needed to detox) and exacerbates stressful emotions, which create emotional toxins in your body. Avoid it during a cleanse.

- Avoid anything canned as much as possible, or with a long list of additives and preservatives. As a general rule, if you can't pronounce one of its ingredients, don't eat it.

- Many of our recipes include nut milks. At least during a cleanse (and if possible all the time), try to prepare them at home. The ones you buy at the grocery store are not fresh, and many times are swimming in unwanted additives.

- Some of our recipes also contain coconut water. Try to find a fresh coconut, cut it, and use that water. Otherwise, there are some brands that sell raw coconut juice without any additives. Pasteurized coconut water is dead food. It probably won't harm you, but it won't nourish you the way raw coconut water does.

BITTER IS BETTER

Do you love sweets? No reason to feel bad about it! In fact, it may mean you're a very evolved human being. Liking this taste is a basic survival strategy, as sweetness is an indicator that what you're eating is not poisonous. Have you ever bitten on a bad almond and thought it tasted wonderfully sweet? Neither have I. When things go bad, they usually become bitter, sometimes overwhelmingly so (in the case of almonds, they taste like actual poison). This is the truth behind most of us frowning at bitter flavors yet going crazy for milder and sweeter ones: we want to avoid toxins that could get us sick or even kill us.

But when it comes to this group of foods, things are more complex than they seem. You know how sometimes the cause of something is also its antidote? That is true in this case, as large portions of bitter foods tend to be toxic, yet in little doses, many of them can actually help our bodies get rid of toxins. Nature never stops finding ways to amaze.

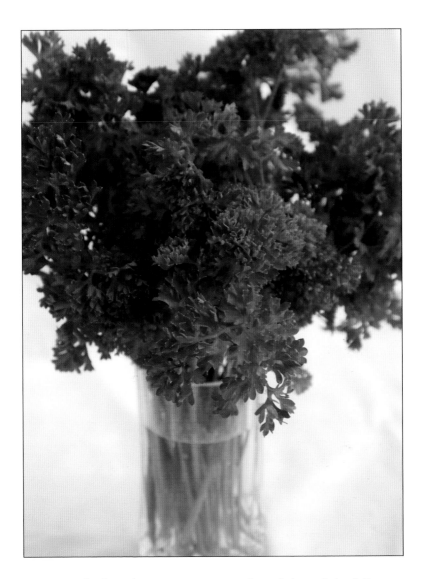

Bitter foods such as watercress, arugula, radish, and dandelion are actually the most detoxifying of all. They stimulate the liver, improve kidney function, regulate blood sugar, and improve nutrient assimilation. When you find them in some of our juices, know that we're not doing it as a cruel joke, but that there's a powerful reason behind it.

BOOSTING UP YOUR JUICES WITH SUPERFOODS

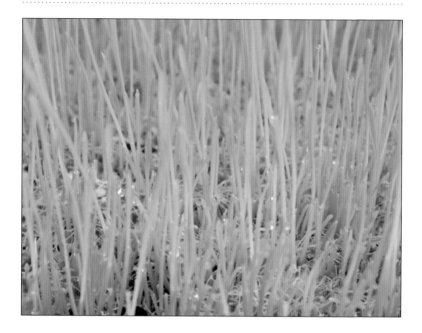

If you walk into a health foods store or the health foods isle of the supermarket, you will find a group of strange-looking ingredients (with even stranger names) that are known as superfoods. These trendy foods owe their cool title to the fact that they have very concentrated doses of certain nutrients. Consuming them can greatly impact your health in many positive ways.

Many of these superfoods are sold as powders or seeds, and the easiest way to consume them is by adding them to juices or smoothies. This makes them a great complement to your detox juicing regime, as several of them will also boost your body's detoxification process, while giving you lots of other fantastic benefits. Some of these food supplements will enhance the taste and texture of your juices, make them more filling, and provide you with massive amounts of energy as well.

We have included these ingredients in some of the juices in the recipe section. However, feel free to add them to as many juices as you want.

Here's a list of our favorites:

- Chia seeds absorb many times their weight in water. When they do this, they secrete a gel that binds toxins and heavy metals, and draws them out of your body. They are neutral in flavor, but will change the texture of your juices and fill you up. Add one teaspoon to your juices, stir, and let them soak for five or ten minutes, until they plump up.
- Chlorella is a green algae with extremely high amounts of chlorophyll (40 times more than wheatgrass!), vitamins, minerals, and trace elements. Just one look at its mind-blowing dark green color is evidence of its richness in nutrients. This sea veggie detoxifies the body from pollutants and heavy metals, purifying the blood and body tissues. The taste is strong and will overpower your juices, but if your priority is health, then you know what to do.
- Cayenne pepper can be added in small quantities to any juice or to water. It is known to remove plaque from the arteries, clean the blood and rebuild its cells, improve circulation, rid the body of bad cholesterol, and eliminate waste.
- Aloe vera is wonderful to have on hand during a cleanse, as it's tasteless and can be blended into any juice. It will neutralize the toxins in the body, stimulate cellular regeneration, and cleanse the colon. To use it, cut a two-inch piece and soak it in water overnight. Separate the gel from the green skin with a knife, and put the gel in the blender with your fresh juice. You can also buy it ready as a gel or juice.
- Coconut oil is one of my favorite ingredients during a cleanse, as it can be added to any juice for instant energy. This antifungal and antibacterial oil was thought to cause heart disease in the past, because it has a saturated fat called lauric acid. It's now been proved that lauric acid is actually very beneficial for health, lowering bad cholesterol and restoring normal thyroid function. This super oil also helps lower blood sugar levels, making it a great complement for sweet fruit juices.
- Flaxseeds can be added to juices both whole and ground, and either way will make them more filling. If you use them whole, they will help you flush out toxins and move your bowel. If you grind them you will absorb all their rich omega-3 oils and their great antioxidant capacity. It's better if you grind your flaxseeds in

the moment to keep all those healthy fats intact. All you need is a coffee grinder and one extra minute.

- Hemp (seeds or powder) is rich in essential fatty acids, and is one of the best protein sources in the plant world. Add hemp to your morning smoothies or juices to feel full and energized throughout the day.
- Maca is an Andean root that belongs to the carrot family. It is known as the Peruvian ginseng for its energizing power. It also helps regulate hormones, and boosts sexual function. Use it sparingly in juices and smoothies—a teaspoon a day is all you need—because its strong flavor can be overwhelming.
- Wheatgrass juice is chock-full of chlorophyll, protein, and vitamin E. Having one shot of this juice is one of the most detoxifying and health-enhancing things you can do, and it's said to add a day to your life. If you put a bit of time and effort, you can juice wheatgrass at home and add it to your juices (you will need a wheatgrass juicer). Otherwise, go to your favorite juice bar and get a fresh wheatgrass shot whenever you can.
- Tahini is the Middle Eastern sesame seed paste added to hummus to give it that creamy texture. Made with raw sesame seeds, it has a thinner consistency than peanut butter and is more bitter. This paste contains all the goodness of sesame seeds in a concentrated form. It's the richest source of calcium you will ever find! Store it in the fridge.
- Spirulina is a mega-healing and detox agent from the ocean. The dark green microalgae is packed with protein, iron, omega-3s, and vitamins B, C, D, A, and E. You either can take it as tablets or add it as powder to your drinks.
- Sacha inchi oil is made of the sacha inchi seed, native to the Peruvian Amazon jungle. This seed, which looks and tastes like a nut, has the highest levels of omega-3 fatty acids in the plant world, making it a powerful anti-inflammatory agent, and a brain, heart, and immune booster. It's important to avoid any kind of heat when consuming its oil, as it is extremely temperature sensitive.

CHAPTER FIVE:
O IS FOR ORGANIC

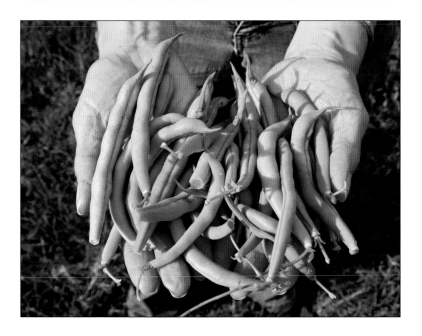

Knowing what organic food represents for your health is an amazing tool that can dramatically lower your exposure to toxins, and can help improve your life and that of those around you.

If you don't know what this is all about, it's okay. We will fix that right away.

Here's the spiel.

THE POISONS IN OUR FOOD

If you've ever had a garden, you will know that sneaky little bugs are always trying to lounge on all kinds of plants, feast on them, and, when they're done, leave them in a less-than-perfect state. This is if some contagious disease doesn't spread from plant to plant first, making them unwelcoming even for insects. To avoid this, you can use chemical substances that will keep all kinds of invaders away, and ensure that you have a beautiful garden.

The same is true when it comes to farming. Conventional agriculture is very efficient at growing humongous amounts of food. To ensure a good crop each time, these big companies make sure their farmers add all kinds of artificial fertilizers, enhancers, and pesticides to the soil and directly to the plants. This is great for them, because it means a bigger and more uniform crop, and, hence, more profit. But when you eat the food that has grown under these conditions you also end up eating all the poisons originally directed at the bugs and diseases, and at creating perfect little fruits and veggies (at least, perfect on the outside) that all look the same.

It always bewilders me to see pictures of farmers spraying their crops in huge astronaut suits to protect them from those poisons. Yet, they consider it okay to put those same poisons that were so harmful for them to breathe, or to put in touch with their skins, inside our bodies. It doesn't make any sense at all, does it?

And this is only half the story.

Where Did the Nutrients Go?

What happens to plants showered with chemical substances at a cellular level is the plant equivalent of us being fed antibiotics. By now you may probably know that antibiotics prescribed to kill bad bacteria in the body also kill the healthy bacteria that keep disease at bay. In the long run, this cure is actually the beginning of new problems, as it taxes our immune system and makes us weaker and more prone to falling sick.

Plants too become weaker when sprayed with chemicals that are meant to protect them. When these plants realize they don't need their own defense mechanisms anymore, they start developing weaker ones. This "immune system" is what contains a lot of the nutrients that we get from plants when we eat them. If the plants don't develop these strengthening nutrients that help keep them healthy, because artificial substances do this for them, we also get less nutrition out of them when we eat them.

In short, plants + chemicals = less nutrition + toxins.

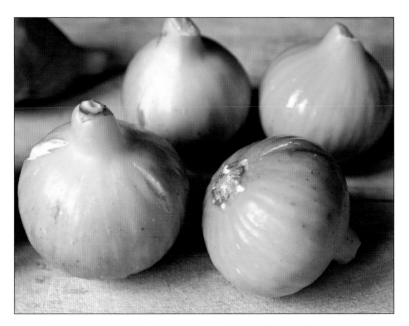

ORGANIC SOUNDS GREAT, BUT NOT EVERYONE CAN AFFORD IT

Organic produce tends to be more expensive than its conventional counterpart, and perhaps you don't think it's worth the extra penny or you plainly cannot afford it. What to do in that case? First of all, don't worry too much. Remember that negative emotions create . . . You guessed it . . . Toxins! There are some simple ways to make organic foods more accessible to you, which is great if you want to eat poison-free foods.

Here's how:

1. Look for seasonal produce. Seasonal foods are more abundant and superior in taste and nutrients. They are also better for your overall health, as your body needs those specific nutrients at the specific time of year when they're available. Organic seasonal produce also tends to be on sale. To plan your juices, check out which fruits and vegetables are in season at any given moment, and then look for the recipes in this book that contain those ingredients

(we've done this for you in the detox programs in Chapter Seven). You can find seasonal produce charts all over the Internet, such as here: http://www.fieldtoplate.com/guide.php.

2. Buy local. Visiting your organic farmers' market is fun, will get you out in the sun, guarantees better nutrition, as less time passes between the farm and your table, and, most importantly, it's easy on your wallet. You can usually get better prices from local farmers than from organic produce that has had to travel from a different continent to your neighborhood's supermarket. Makes sense, right?

3. Be curious and talk to your farmer. Sometimes foods are not labeled as organic because labeling them entails a long and expensive bureaucratic process that farmers cannot always afford. You can talk to your local farmers and find out if they spray their products with chemicals or not. You may be pleasantly surprised, and you may gain a few new friends too.

4. Join a co-op. You may have to pay to join a food cooperative, but once you're a part of it you can start getting great-quality food

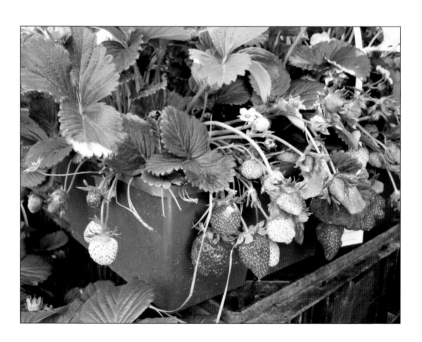

at discounted prices. As a member, you may need to work a few hours a month in exchange for the benefits you get, but you will end up saving so much on food that doing it will be worth every minute of your time.

5. Pay attention to the Dirty Dozen, and chill out when it comes to the Clean Fifteen.

The Dirty Dozen

Although we recommend you try to get organic whenever possible, if it's unavailable to you for whatever reason, there are a couple lists that will take you a long way in cleaning up your food act. There are twelve crops you should be suspicious about, as they are the most heavily sprayed and hence the most toxic to your system. Some people avoid them altogether unless they're organic, yet others believe the health benefits of eating them will override the negative effects of the pesticides that have been used to grow them. All we can say is try your very best to get these in their organic variety. And at the very least, clean them particularly well and peel them if they have skin.

These include:

- Apples
- Celery
- Cherry tomatoes
- Cucumbers
- Grapes
- Hot peppers
- Nectarines (imported)
- Peaches
- Potatoes
- Spinach
- Strawberries
- Bell peppers

The Environmental Working Group, which tailors this list, also calls attention to kale, collard greens, summer squash, and zucchini, as they test positive for two highly toxic pesticides.

The Clean Fifteen

Luckily, there's a happier list of foods that are considered safe (or safer) even if they are not organic. This is usually the case with fruits and veggies that have thick skins to protect their pulp from any outside contamination, or that don't need to be heavily sprayed.

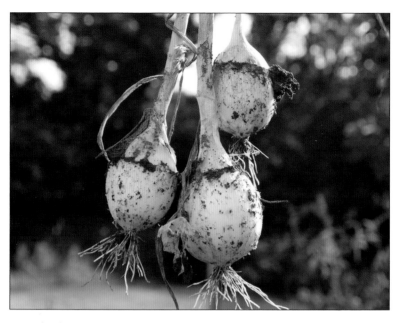

This list includes:

- Sweet potatoes
- Sweet peas
- Pineapples
- Papayas
- Onions
- Mushrooms
- Mangoes
- Kiwis
- Grapefruit
- Eggplants
- Sweet corn
- Cantaloupe
- Avocados
- Cabbage
- Asparagus

If you can afford to buy only some organic produce, you can focus on being paranoid about the Dirty Dozen. Your diet won't be perfectly clean and 100 percent the way nature intended it to be, but hey, let's not let perfect get in the way of pretty good.

CLEANING YOUR VEGGIES

Whether you buy organic fruits and veggies or not, all your produce should be cleaned before eating to remove toxins, which include chemicals, dirt, and bacteria. Your body needs to work extra hard to clean out all of these freeloaders if you don't make time for this before you put the food in your mouth. Why give your body that extra load instead of letting it focus on cleaning what's already stored in there from too much fun in the past? All it will take is a few minutes, some salt, and half a lemon.

Jay Kordich, known as "the father of juicing," has been juicing away for the past sixty-something years, and his amazing health and stamina at the age of ninety is a testament to the power of these drinks. In their blog, Jay and his wife Linda recommend you clean all your fruits and veggies by filling your kitchen sink with cold water, adding four tablespoons of salt and the juice of half a lemon, and soaking the fruits and vegetables for five to ten minutes; two to three minutes for leafy greens, and one to two minutes for berries. When the time is up, rinse well under cold running water, and go about your juicing business.

Since we are trying to get you the least exposure to toxins as possible during your cleanse, we would like to take their washing instructions one step further, and recommend that you use filtered water whenever possible when washing your veggies. This way your juicing ingredients won't end up covered in heavy metals, pesticides, and other substances added to tap water, such as chlorine, which kills harmful bugs but also your intestinal flora. It's as easy as buying a water filter, and making sure you change the filter as recommended in the package. If this is too time consuming, however, don't worry too much about it, as the benefits of juicing will outweigh the negative effects of consuming a little bit of unfiltered tap water.

CHAPTER SIX:
RECIPES

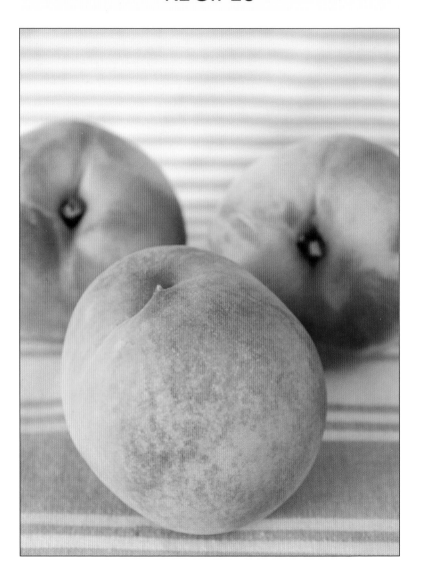

WHAT YOU WILL NEED:

- Juicer
- Blender
- Measuring cups
- Measuring spoons
- Knife

- Chopping board
- Water filter (optional)
- Colander
- Cocktail shaker (optional)
- Vegetable peeler (optional)

A few tips before you get started:

1. Wash everything first.
2. If you're using organic fruits and veggies, you can keep the skin of some fruits and veggies on. The obvious skins to avoid are kiwi, mango, grapefruit, etc. Use common sense here. If you're not using organic ingredients, peel all the fruits and veggies that have a skin.
3. Cut your ingredients in chunks that will fit into your juicer. For smoothies, cut them in smaller chunks.
4. When making smoothies, use the blender at low speed so the heat it creates doesn't destroy some of the important enzymes in your fruits and veggies.
5. When a recipe calls for nut milks, pomegranate juice, coconut water, and the like, make your best effort to get them fresh. Commercial versions have been pasteurized at high temperatures and are devoid of many of the amazing nutrients that abound in the fresh product.
6. Drink your juices and smoothies as soon as you make them whenever possible, to get the best nutrition out of them. If absolutely necessary, keep in the fridge for up to a day in an airtight glass container filled all the way to the top (mason jars work well). If your time is very constrained, you can make several juices at once, and freeze them immediately. Thaw in the fridge individually, when you're ready to drink them.
7. You can keep the skin on when juicing organic lemons, limes, and oranges if you want. However, be mindful of the taste and how you feel. They may turn some juices too bitter for you, and the orange peel's natural oils may cause upset stomach in some people.
8. Keep your veggies in separate plastic bags in the fridge, and don't

wash them until you use them. This way they will last longer without going limp. As a general rule, fruits and veggies are easier to juice when they are fresh and "crunchy," leafy greens and herbs in particular.

9. Herbs can be stored in the fridge with the stalks inside a glass with water (just like you would do with flowers), and the leaves covered with a plastic bag.

10. These recipes are not set in stone. Add the flavors you enjoy, and leave out those that don't work for you. The portions will also vary depending on the size and quality of the fruits and veggies you buy, and the juicer you have. So feel free to adjust the amounts the recipes call for to get a portion of juice that feels right for you.

11. The less sweet your juice is, the better it is for you. It's okay if you have to start with the sweeter juices, but try to slowly work your way to a ratio of 3 to 1 (three vegetable portions for every fruit portion).

12. There are several types of juicers, and any of them work well to get you started in juicing. However, there are a few types that perform better than others: starting with a twin-gear juicer, followed by a masticating juicer, and lastly, a centrifugal juicer. They also tend to be priced according to quality, so keep that in mind if money is an issue.

BASICS

- Health Nut (a.k.a. Nut Milk)
- Lemon-aid
- Spice of Life
- Super Seed Me (a.k.a. Seed Milk)
- Hawaiian Elixir (a.k.a. Pineapple Water)

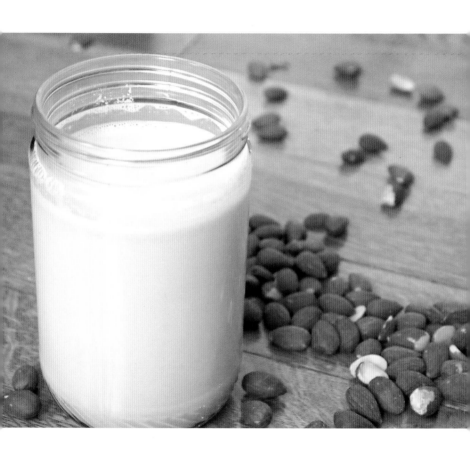

Health Nut (a.k.a. Nut Milk)

Makes 2½–3 cups

In the past few years, dairy has been demonized by the health food industry, and milk alternatives have been on the rise. However, most of the substitutes that well-intentioned people have adopted as part of their new and "improved" diets have scary-named chemicals listed in their ingredients, and are definitely not what we would call fresh. So why not make them from scratch instead and get all their wonderful benefits? It's easy peasy and your body will notice the difference.

1 cup nuts, raw unsalted (you can pick any of these: almonds, pecans, hazelnuts, Brazil nuts, walnuts)
2 cups water

- Put the nuts in a bowl, cover with water, and soak overnight.
- In the morning, drain the water and rinse the nuts.
- If they can be peeled (like almonds), it's better if you do it, as the skin is hard to digest. The peel should come off easily.
- Process the nuts in a blender with 2 cups water, until they have completely liquefied.
- Pass through a sieve, pressing the solids that stay at the bottom with the back of a spoon, until no more liquid drips out of it.
- Refrigerate in an airtight container for up to 3 days, and stir well before using, because the tiny nut particles tend to accumulate at the bottom.
- Don't throw out the fiber you get when you drain the milk! See the tip box on page 53 for ideas on what to do with it.

When you include nut milk in your juices and smoothies, its protein helps stabilize your blood sugar levels even if you add sweet fruits to the preparation. Due to its high fat content, it takes longer to digest and keeps you full for many hours. This is why we love adding this wonderful milk to our morning drinks.

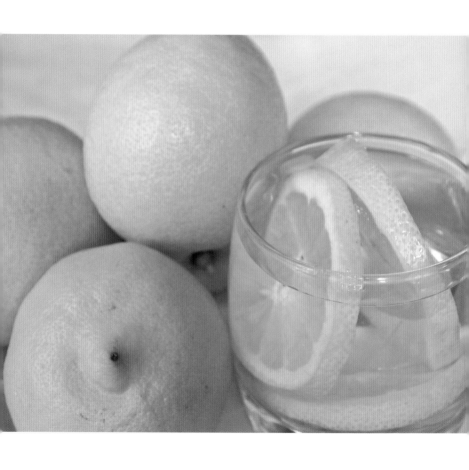

Lemon-aid

Makes 1 glass

It is common knowledge that drinking warm water with lemon upon rising helps purify the body. This is a great practice to adopt and turn into a daily ritual, and with practice, it will become automatic, just like brushing your teeth or having breakfast. If you want to take this one step further, add an extra lemon each day, for a whole week, and then start taking out a lemon a day, for another week.

1 glass water (warm or at room temperature)
1 lemon

- ◆ Squeeze the lemon into the water and drink immediately.
- ◆ Bonus: While you drink it, thank the water for purifying, healing, and energizing every cell of your body.

It may sound like a contradiction, but lemon, the fruit that makes your face twitch with its acidity, has an alkalizing effect on the body. When this is drunk first thing in the morning, it flushes out toxins and helps restore the slightly alkaline pH of your blood.

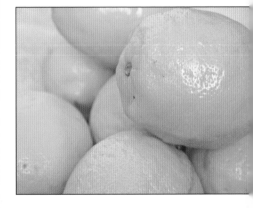

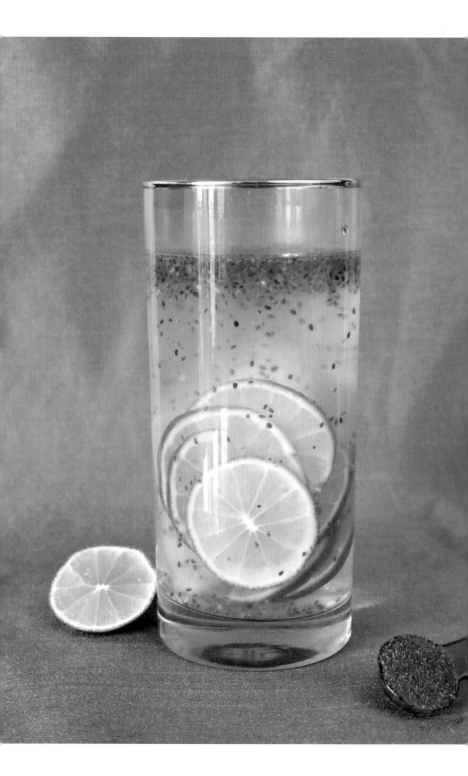

Spice of Life

Makes 1 glass

This spicy water is an upgraded version of the powerfully cleansing water with lemon. All you need to do is add some warming and energizing ginger, a fiber megadose in the form of chia seeds, and a sprinkling of cayenne pepper to wake up your body's circulatory system.

1-inch piece ginger, finely chopped
1 tablespoon chia seeds
Juice of 1 lime
A pinch of ground cayenne pepper

- Put the ginger in a pan with 2 cups of water, and bring to a boil.
- Let it cool for a few minutes, and once it's lukewarm, remove the ginger, transfer to a glass, and add the chia seeds. Stir and soak for 5 minutes.
- Add the lime juice, and sprinkle with cayenne pepper.
- Stir and serve.

Lemons and limes are an important component of most juices in this book for many reasons. For one, they stimulate your taste buds, making any drink more enjoyable. They also bring down the bitterness and strong taste of the most robust veggies, such as kale, watercress, and wheatgrass. Their vitamin C content is exceptional, and if this wasn't enough, they slow down the oxidizing process in your juices (just like they do in your body), keeping them from turning an unappealing brown.

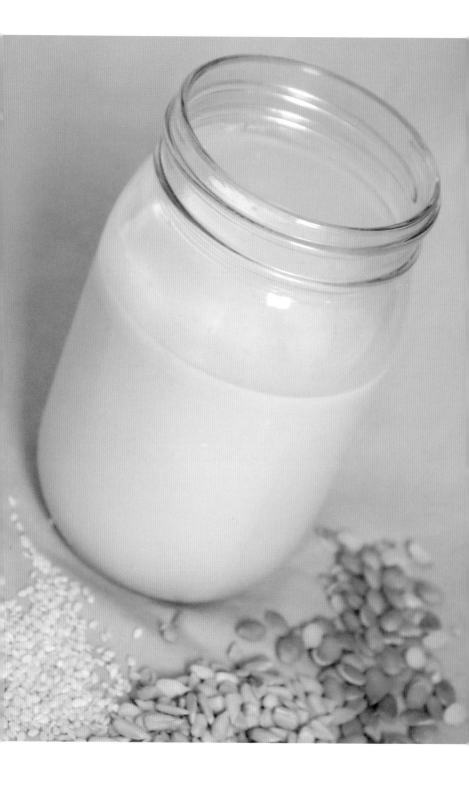

Super Seed Me (a.k.a. Seed Milk)

Makes 3 cups

Nowadays it's easy to find alternative milks wherever you go. Rice, soy, almond . . . you name it. But I'm always thinking of ways to take my nutrition one step further and to have fun in the kitchen. That is how this super seed milk was created. Instead of munching on these seeds when you're hungry, why not drink a refreshing glass of milk made from them?

⅓ cup sesame seeds
⅓ cup pumpkin seeds
⅓ cup sunflower seeds
2 cups water

- Soak the seeds overnight in a bowl of water.
- In the morning, drain the water, and then process the seeds in a blender with 2 cups water, until you have a smooth liquid.
- Pass through a strainer, and press the remaining solids with a spoon to get all the water out of them.
- Store this milk in an airtight container in the fridge, for up to 3 days.

When you make seed or nut milk you may be left with quite a bit of fiber after blending and straining it. Why throw it away? You can use it in bread or muffin recipes, add it to all kinds of smoothies, sprinkle it over your breakfast or salads, or even mix it with honey and yogurt for a wonderful homemade face and body scrub.

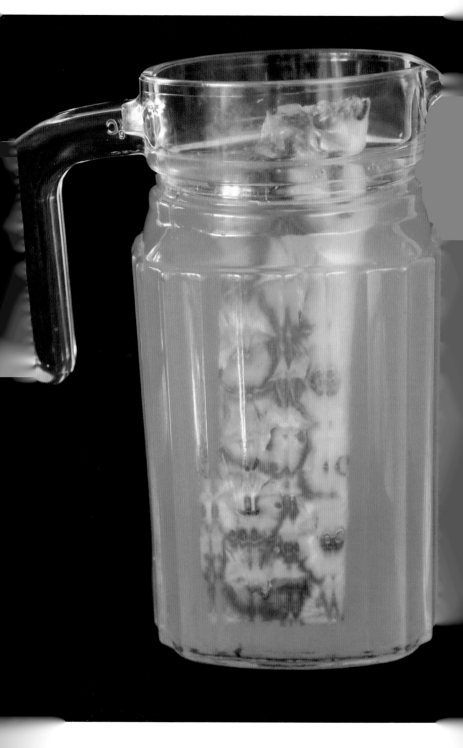

Hawaiian Elixir (a.k.a. Pineapple Water)

Makes 4 cups

This flavorful water is a dieter's dream: spicy, slightly sweet yet sugar free, and highly diuretic. Use it as the base for smoothies, or make it without the spices and grab a glass whenever you're thirsty to replace regular water (those who claim they don't drink water because it's tasteless will be thankful for this recipe). This is a great way to use pineapple peels instead of throwing them away.

1 organic pineapple (skin only)
1 cinnamon stick
4 allspice berries
2 cloves
5 cups water

- Clean the pineapple peel by scrubbing it with a brush under hot running water.
- Combine the pineapple peel, cinnamon, allspice, cloves, and 5 cups water in a saucepan.
- Bring to a boil over medium heat and simmer for about 30 minutes. Turn off the heat and cool.
- Strain, discarding the solids. Transfer the pineapple water to a jar and keep refrigerated or at room temperature.

Forget sugary drinks or artificially flavored water. When cooking corn, save the water and drink it during the day for a diuretic effect. The cooking water of potatoes is traditionally used for kidney problems, particularly for stones or sediments. Mix and match these with fruits and spices to create your own trademark drinks.

SUPER POWER GREENS

- Cool as a Cucumber
- Green Is In
- Holy Kale
- Simply Green
- Sweetchini
- Green Up
- Healthy Mary
- Green Raw-volution
- Thin like an Asparagus
- Broccolini Genie

- All You Need Is Kale
- Twist and Sprout
- I Love Radishes
- Better than a V8
- Scarborough Fair
- The Sweet Smell of Success
- Pear-fect Health
- Berry Good
- Serious Business
- Heart Chakra

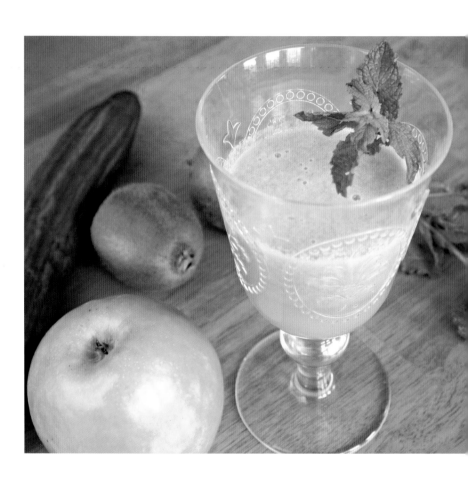

Cool as a Cucumber

Makes 1 glass

This juice is the epitome of coolness thanks to the light and refreshing effect of cucumbers and mint. Serve it over ice (or turn it into a slushy with crushed ice), and you have the secret weapon to survive any summer heat wave untouched.

½ cucumber
1 Granny Smith apple
1 kiwi, peeled
3 sprigs mint
1 cup parsley
½ lemon

♦ Process all the ingredients in a juicer and serve.

Mint's menthol oils are a natural cure for indigestion, stomach ulcers, and food poisoning. They also help clear a congested head and chest in allergic people, or during colds and flu processes. You can grow this garden herb indoors, and cut it right before using so it's fresh as the morning dew when you juice it. You can't get more "local" than that!

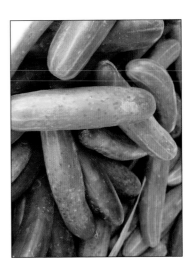

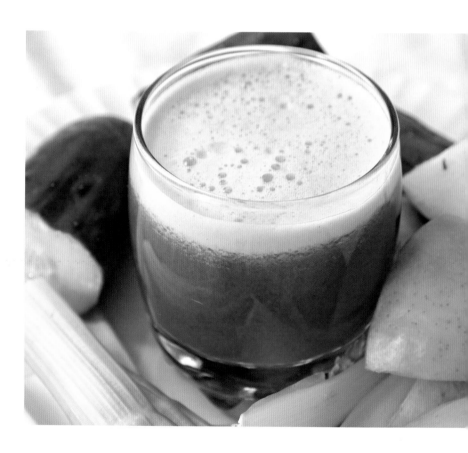

Green Is In

Makes 1 glass

If I had to recommend just one juice from our repertoire, this simple green recipe would perhaps be the winner. This drink is like a canvas for all the other fruits, vegetables, and superfoods lying around in your kitchen. And yes, you can think of yourself as the juice artist! Enjoy it as it is, or add whatever your body yearns for, making it new and exciting every time you drink it.

½ cucumber
½ Granny Smith apple
2 celery ribs
½–1 heart of romaine
1–2 cups spinach, chard, or kale

 ◆ Juice all the ingredients and serve.

Green apples have a lower glycemic index (GI) than most fruits, and that's why they're a great alternative to sweeten your juices. Including ingredients with a low GI in your juices will keep your blood sugar levels stable, which translates into fewer cravings, better mood, and higher levels of energy throughout the whole day.

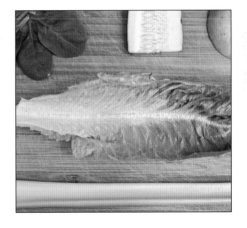

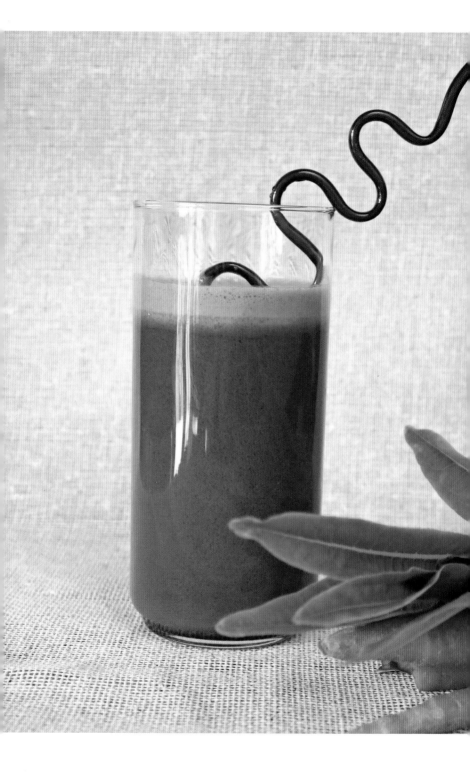

Holy Kale

Makes 1 glass

This juice is a great way to stock up on robust leafy greens without even noticing it. It has a pleasant parsley flavor with a lightly salted celery touch, and the sweetness of the carrots and apple are also present in every drop. Kale, however, goes almost unnoticed.

1–2 carrots
2 kale leaves
4 lettuce leaves
½ cup parsley
½ Granny Smith apple
2 celery ribs
½ lemon

- ◆ Process all the ingredients in a juicer and serve.

Carrots are ideal for juicing because they have a high water content and add their characteristic sweetness to any recipe. They will also strengthen your eyes and give your skin a beautiful golden tan in the summer that will be the envy of many. So stock up on them!

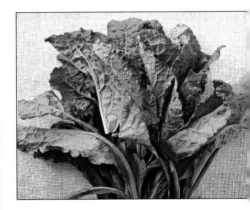

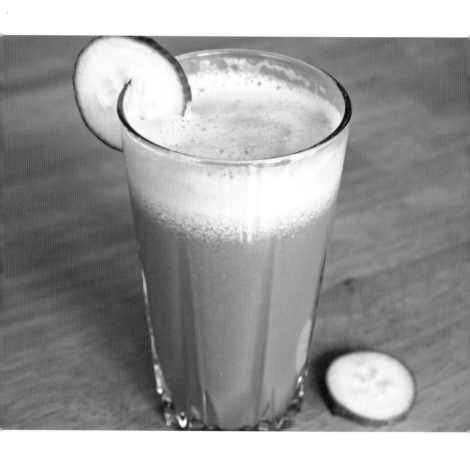

Simply Green

Makes 1 glass

This is a much healthier pick-me-up than most commercial cereal bars or coffee. Notice that the recipe doesn't include any sweet fruits or veggies, which makes it your blood sugar's dream juice. A glass of it will alkalize your body, filling it with oxygen and giving your cells many of the essential nutrients they crave.

½ cucumber
3 celery ribs
2 cups spinach
½–1 lime or lemon

+ Process all the ingredients in a juicer and serve.

This juice is so low in calories and sugar that you can drink it throughout the day to keep yourself hydrated. If you drink it often, it's better if you rotate the leafy greens and don't stick to the spinach every single time (chard, lettuce, and kale are other good alternatives). You can have too much of a good thing, and overdoing the same dark leafy greens all the time can have a toxic effect on some people.

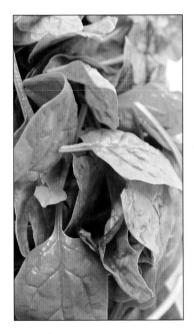

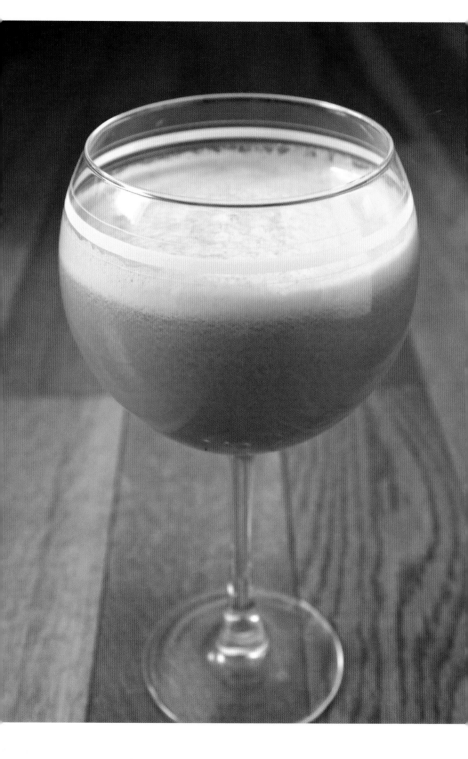

Sweetchini

Makes 1 glass

Surprisingly sweet, despite having only one sweet fruit listed among its ingredients, when you drink this you will be able to relax and enjoy the experience, while the juice does the rest.

2 cups green beans
½–1 zucchini
½ lemon
1 apple
1 cup parsley

* Juice all the ingredients and serve.

Herbs can be difficult to juice in certain juicers. One solution is to stop the juicer and throw a few pieces of fruit or veggies in it. Add a handful of herbs, and top with more fruits or veggies. Only then, turn the juicer on and start pressing. When sandwiched this way, tiny leaves and sprouts are more likely to yield juice.

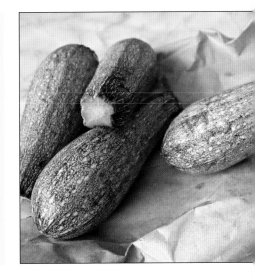

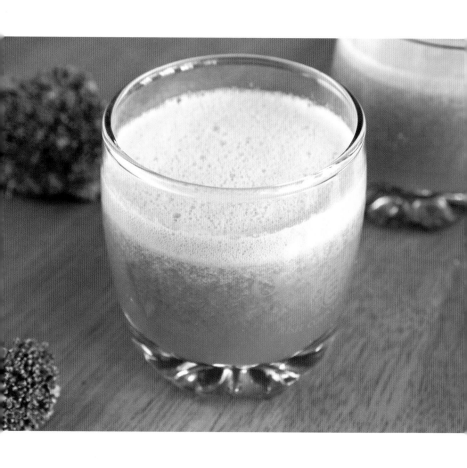

Green Up

Makes 1 glass

Broccoli doesn't have an unpleasant or strong flavor when added to juices. In fact, it has a slightly sweet effect. This sulfur-rich veggie helps the liver detoxification pathways work properly. Don't be shy and use every part of it: florets, stems, and leaves.

1 cup broccoli
1 Granny Smith apple
1 cup pineapple
2 cups spinach
½-inch piece ginger, peeled

- ♦ Put all the ingredients in a juicer, process, and serve.

A small amount of ginger in your juice can enhance many flavors and conceal others that you're not crazy about. Ayurveda recommends chewing on a piece of ginger before every meal to turn on your digestive fire. Chinese medicine, on the other hand, uses dried ginger for very powerful purposes, such as awakening those who have fallen into a coma. Yes, that kind of powerful.

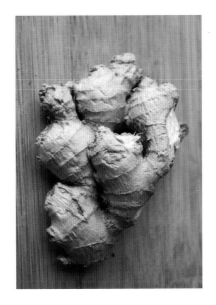

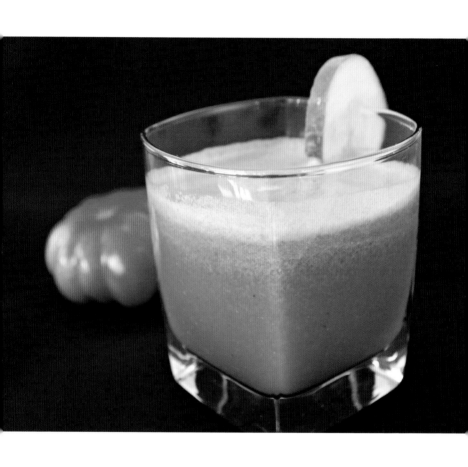

Healthy Mary

Makes 1 glass

Forget hangovers, and welcome younger-looking skin, a slimmer body, more energy, and all-around awesomeness. This low-calorie savory juice will make you feel like you're always on vacation, sipping Bloody Marys in the middle of the day, but without any of the negative effects. Cheers to that!

½ bell pepper
½ cucumber
½ zucchini
1 tomato
1 cup lettuce
½–1 lime
Dash of cayenne pepper

- Process the bell pepper, cucumber, zucchini, tomato, lettuce, and lime in a juicer.
- Add a sprinkling of cayenne pepper, stir, and serve.
- You can put a celery stick in the glass for a real virgin Bloody Mary effect.

Legend has it that bell peppers are fabulous for the skin, and adding just a little piece of them to juices will give you a smooth and glowing complexion. Worth giving it a shot, don´t you think?

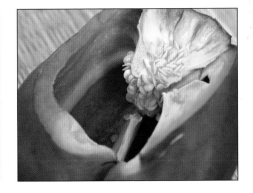

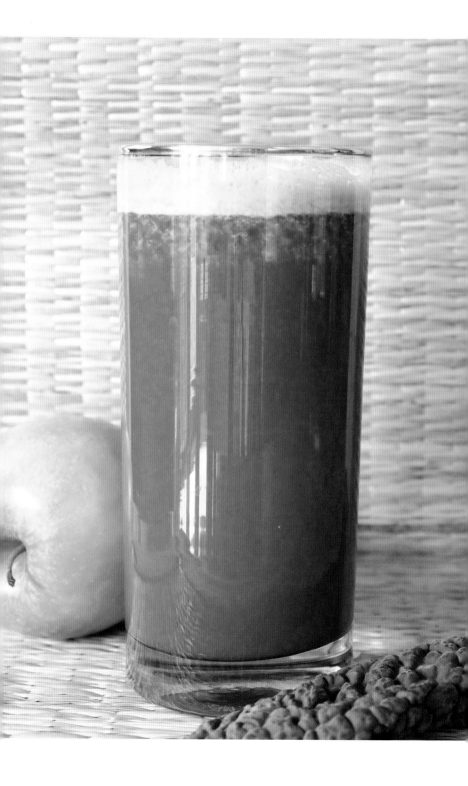

Green Raw-volution

Makes 1 glass

Some health experts believe that the best time to have a replenishing drink like this is first thing in the morning. When you wake up, after several hours of natural "fasting" while you're sleeping, your body doesn't have any half-digested food blocking the road. A powerful green juice like this will breeze right into your bloodstream and cells.

½ apple
½ orange
½ cucumber
1 cup kale
2 celery ribs
1 tablespoon chia seeds

- Juice all the fruits and veggies.
- Add the chia seeds, stir, and let them soak for 5 to 10 minutes.

If you don't use organic limes, lemons, or oranges, just squeeze them over your juices instead of going through the hassle of peeling them to pass them through the juicer. And don't forget the strainer! You don't want those sneaky little seeds falling into your pure and sparkling glass of juice.

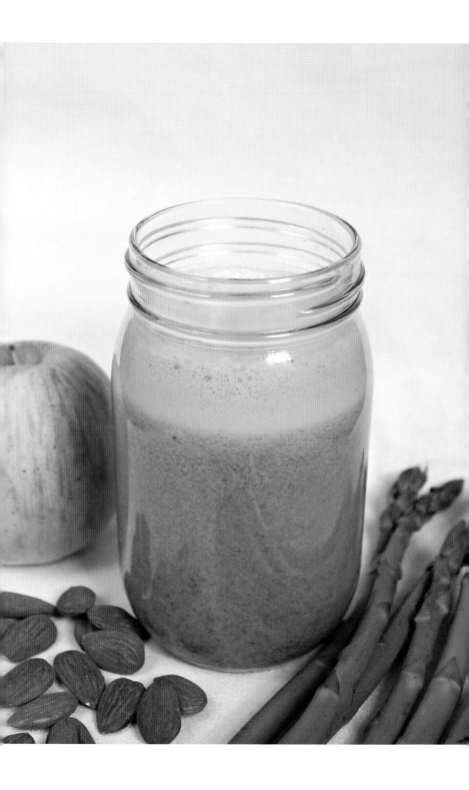

Thin like an Asparagus

Makes 1 glass

Nature has a way of showing us the benefit behind everything it provides in very obvious ways. Walnuts have the shape of a brain, and are particularly good for it too. Beets are red like blood, and cleanse and enrich our own. Asparagus are thin and long, and I don't know about you, but for me it's not a coincidence that they're also a natural weight-loss food.

1 apple
10 asparagus spears
½ zucchini
½ cucumber
½ lemon
1 teaspoon almond butter (optional)

- Juice the apple, asparagus, zucchini, cucumber, and lemon.
- Process this juice in a blender together with the almond butter.

Asparagus can be pricey if bought out of season, so if money is an issue, try to reserve this juice for the time of year when they're more abundant and their price goes down a bit. The wonderful news is that they're usually in full bloom during spring, which is the perfect time to do a cleanse. Asparagus juice protects the liver when drinking alcohol, and is a great hangover cure.

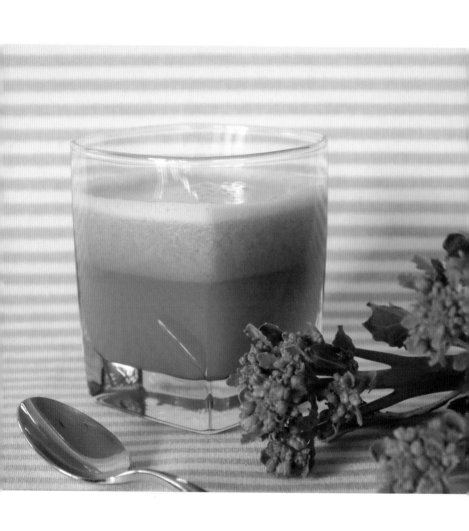

Broccolini Genie

Makes 1 glass

Juicing is simple: if it's green, you can be certain that it's good for you. But don't be misled into thinking that all green juices are the same and, hence, boring. There are all kinds of combinations you can come up with to bring some excitement into them every time. Broccolini is one of those unconventional options that will also help eliminate unwanted contaminants from your body.

1 cup broccolini (florets and stems)
½ cucumber
4 celery ribs
1 ripe pear
½–1 lemon

◆ Juice all the ingredients and serve.

When you juice broccoli, broccolini, or broccoli rabe, make sure you use the stalks and leaves too. People are too fast at throwing away the less attractive parts of fruits and veggies, unbeknownst to the fact that these are also packed with nutrients, sometimes even more so than the beautiful pulp or florets. This family of veggies shouldn't be juiced every single day, as they can become toxic if consumed too often.

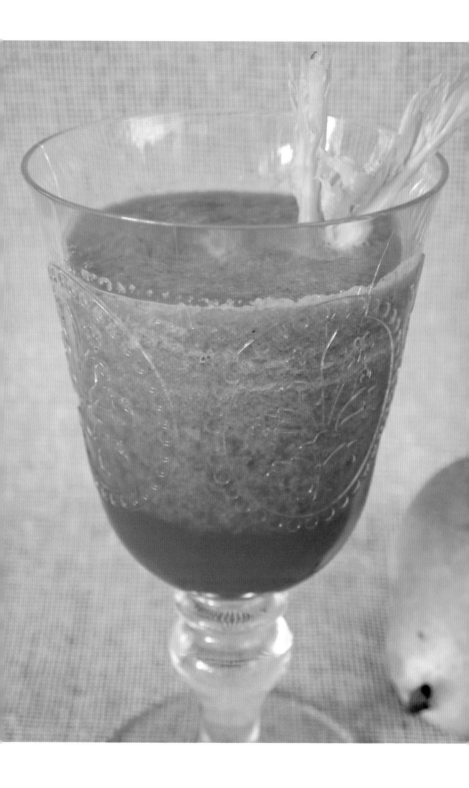

All You Need Is Kale

Makes 1 glass

Kale is all the rage these days because its dark leaves are fantastic at maintaining the beauty of your skin and the strength of your bones, at detoxifying your blood, and at building muscle. If you think you're not getting enough protein to support you after a workout, kale is all you need.

4 kale leaves
1–2 pears
½–1 lime
2 celery ribs
½ cucumber

- ◆ Process all the ingredients in a juicer and serve.

At the beginning of your juicing career, before your palate gets used to greener flavors, we recommend adding pears or apples to your green juices. Once you're ready, you can leave them out of these recipes if you want, or lower their dose.

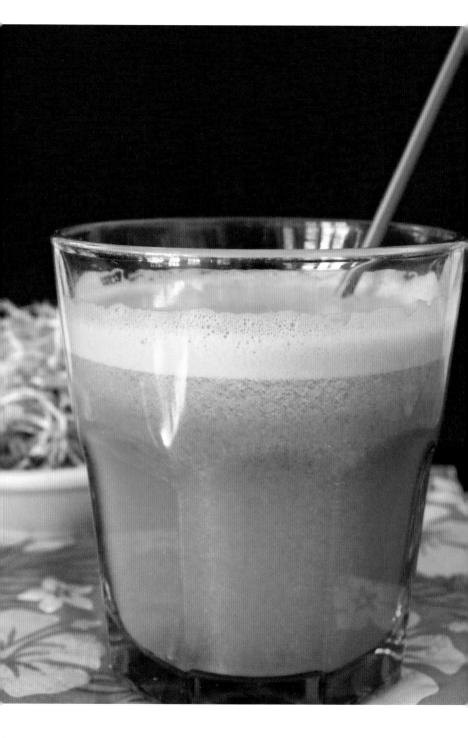

Twist and Sprout

Makes 1 glass

Sprouts have more enzymes than most other foods, and inviting them to your table is the smartest decision you can make on your road toward better health. Think of them as babies: brand new, spotless, and abundant in life force. The vibrant piquancy of broccoli sprouts brings all that and more to this juice.

½ cucumber
3 celery ribs
1 apple
1 cup broccoli sprouts

● Juice all the ingredients and serve.

Broccoli sprouts have a peppery flavor that resembles watercress, radishes, or mustard greens. The apple's gentle sweetness brings this assertiveness down a notch, but if you are looking for something milder try sunflower or alfalfa sprouts. Juice your sprouts sandwiched between the other ingredients to get more juice out of them.

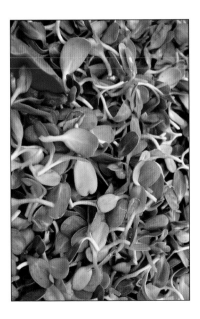

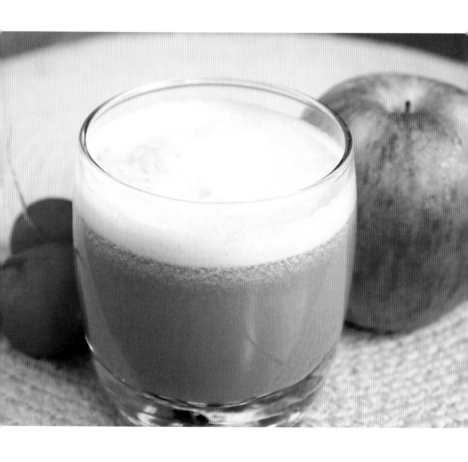

I Love Radishes

Makes 1 glass

Why stop at juicing sweet ingredients when you can also enjoy the pungency that radishes bring to every juice? These cute little veggies will help your liver become your body's worker of the month by providing many essential enzymes for its appropriate functioning. You can experiment with different kinds of radishes, such as daikon radish or black radish.

1 cup zucchini
1 Granny Smith apple
1 small radish
1 cup broccoli
Juice of ½ lemon

- ◆ Juice the first four ingredients.
- ◆ Squeeze in the lemon juice and serve.

If you go to the store or market and can't find the exact ingredients a recipe calls for, don't sweat it. It's easy to vary the ingredients in most juices. Here, for example, you can use cucumber or summer squash instead of zucchini, pear instead of apple, and lime or orange instead of lemon.

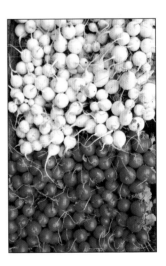

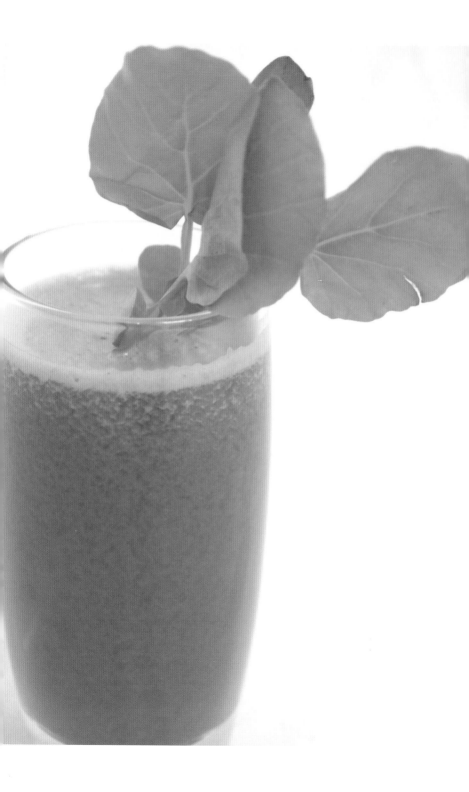

Better than a V8

Makes 1 glass

The idea behind V8 is good: getting a large array of vegetables in a can. But it doesn't come close to drinking a glass of freshly pressed, living juice. This recipe shares some of the ingredients in V8, such as watercress, spinach, celery, and carrots, and has some new ones that we use to counteract the bitterness of watercress.

½ cup watercress
1 cup spinach
2 celery ribs
½ cucumber
1 carrot
1 ripe pear
½–1 Granny Smith apple
½–1 lemon

◆ Juice all the ingredients and serve.

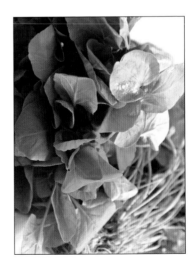

If you run away from bitter flavors, start with just a half cup of watercress, and build up your tolerance to one cup. There's a reason why bitters are included in detox juices: they are the most beneficial foods for the liver. If the taste is still too much for you, add another lemon to the recipe.

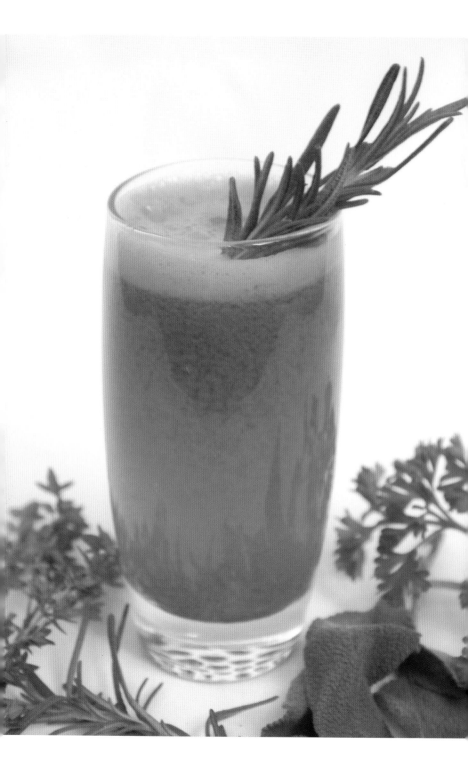

Scarborough Fair

Makes 1 glass

It was hard to resist the temptation of making a juice inspired by one of my favorite songs, Simon and Garfunkel's "Scarborough Fair," especially as my mom and I listened to it a million times while we were writing this book. Learning about the blood-cleansing properties of herbs was the perfect excuse to indulge my playful side and prepare this juice with a sound track. The green liquid that came out was sweet, harmonious, and soothing. Just like the song.

½ cucumber
½ heart of romaine
1 Granny Smith apple
1 cup parsley
2 sprigs sage
2 sprigs rosemary
2 sprigs thyme

- Juice all the ingredients and serve.

If you have a green thumb, growing your own herbs at home is a great time and space investment. These plants are anti-inflammatory, antioxidant, and antimicrobial, and they improve brain function and lower blood sugar levels in diabetics. Wow.

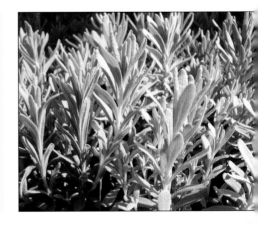

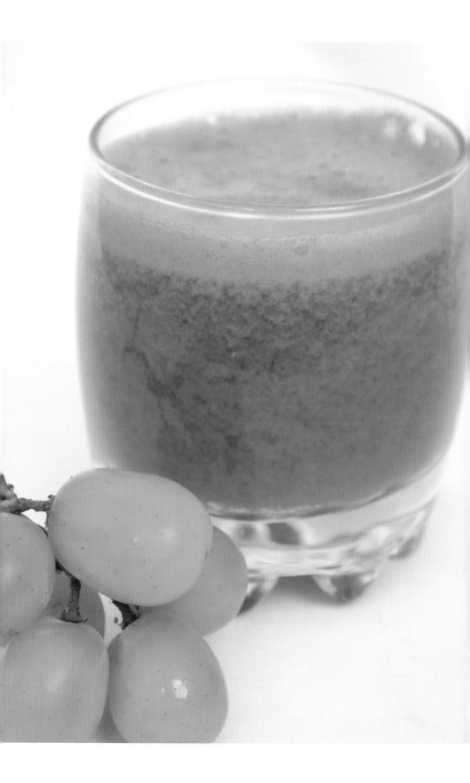

The Sweet Smell of Success

Makes 1 glass

This aromatic juice is one of my favorites, thanks to the nutty and peppery arugula. Green tea, grapes, and lemon bring bucketfuls of antioxidants to the mix, and a perfect balance of sweetness and acidity to the pungent leaves. A recipe for detox success.

½ cup green tea
1 cup arugula
2 cups green grapes
½–1 lemon

- ◆ Make the green tea and let it cool.
- ◆ Juice the arugula, grapes, and lemon.
- ◆ Combine the juice with the green tea.

Many herbs have detoxifying properties, so you can replace green tea with herbal teas. If you want to do this, consider replacing it with dandelion tea, made from the liver-enhancing wonder-leaf.

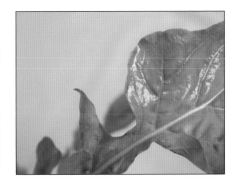

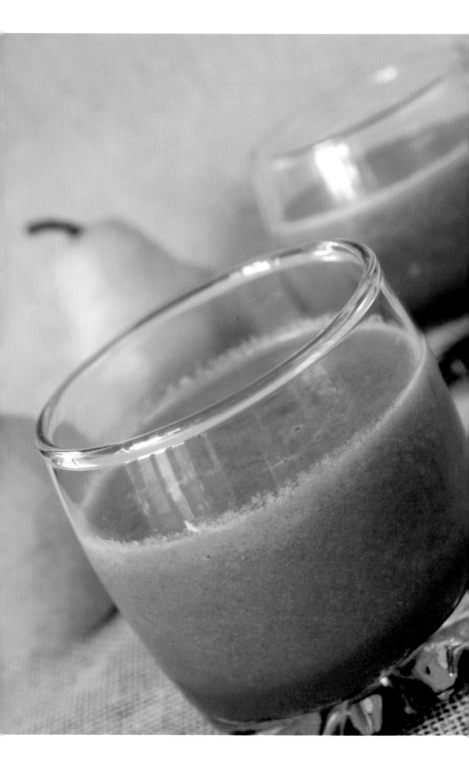

Pear-fect Health

Makes 1 glass

Your body will love this creamy juice, which can be considered hypoallergenic thanks to its main ingredient: pear. With its awesome antioxidant and antibacterial properties, this sweet fruit is safe for everyone, including those who suffer from allergies. This makes it ideal for a detox program, as it will give your system a rest from constantly fighting all kinds of allergens out of your system.

2 ripe pears
2 cups spinach
½-inch piece ginger, peeled
½–1 lime
½ cucumber

- ◆ Juice all the ingredients and serve.

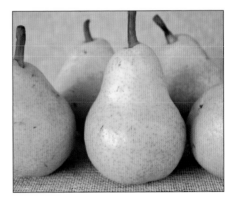

When you buy pears at the farmers' market or grocery store, they will most likely be hard. Keep them on your kitchen counter until they soften, and once they do, consume them within a day or two or they'll quickly go bad.

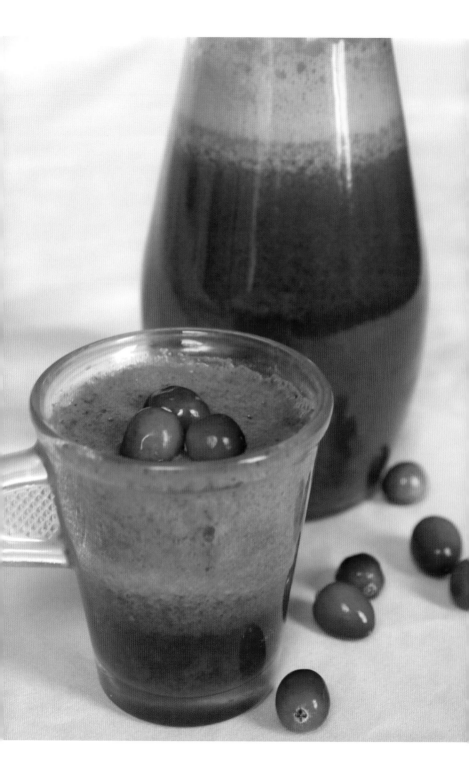

Berry Good

Makes 1 glass

Cranberries are not the easiest fruits to include in your diet, because of their incomparably tart taste. When juiced, however, their taste can be easily balanced with other fruits and vegetables, allowing you to get a concentrated dose of their miraculous health benefits in one glass.

1 cup cranberries
1 apple
2 celery ribs
1 cup spinach
½ cucumber
½ cup cilantro

- Process all the ingredients in a juicer and serve.

Cranberries are nature's solution for urinary tract infections, many of which can be completely cured simply by drinking their juice. If you are taking blood thinners, however, you should avoid drinking cranberry juice, as it can raise the blood levels of these drugs and become dangerous.

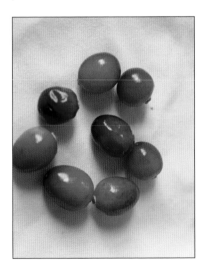

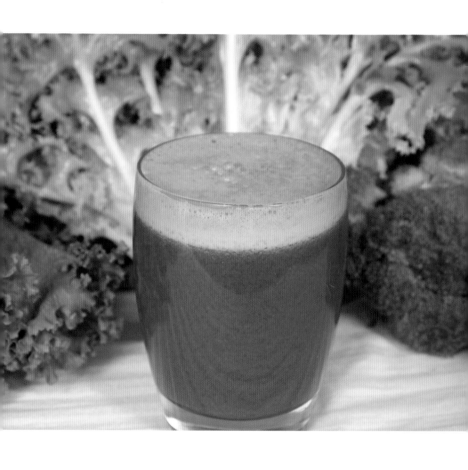

Serious Business

Makes 1 glass

This drink has the exact taste one would expect from a green juice: mild, slightly sweet, with a hint of spice. The peppery flavor is given by mustard greens, a leafy green that we haven't used nearly as much as we should have in this book, because its taste may be too strong for many people. This juice, however, shows how to do it right, enhancing its flavor instead of overpowering it.

½ cucumber
½ cup broccoli
½ Granny Smith apple
2 celery ribs
½ cup spinach
1 cup escarole
1 mustard green leaf

+ Process all the ingredients in a juicer and serve.

The strong personality of mustard greens matches their strong healing power. They lower cholesterol (especially when cooked), and are rich in phytonutrients that help prevent cancer. They are kick-ass detoxifying and anti-inflammatory agents, and they are also full of antioxidants.

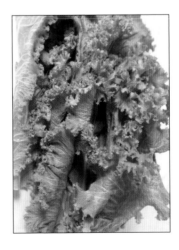

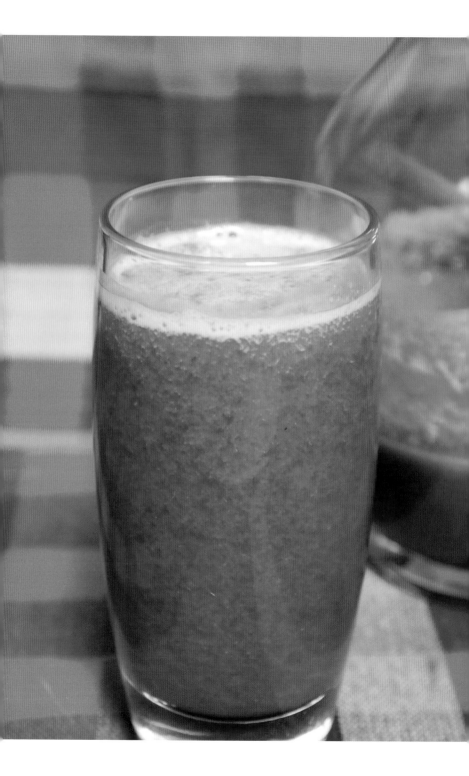

Heart Chakra

Makes 1 glass

The heart chakra is known to be the energetic center of our immune system. It also happens to be green, and is enhanced by any contact with green colors. No wonder green juices are so good for health! Whenever you need to heal any part of your body, you can concentrate on your heart center, and imagine green light being sent from there to the affected area.

2 mustard green leaves
2 kiwis, peeled
½ heart of romaine
½ zucchini
1 cup broccoli
½ lemon
½ cup blueberries

- ◆ Process all the ingredients in a juicer and serve.

Romaine lettuce increases the vitamin and mineral content of juices and smoothies. This leafy veggie should be your best friend if you're looking to lose weight, and you can have as much as you want because its calories are few.

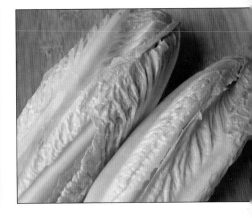

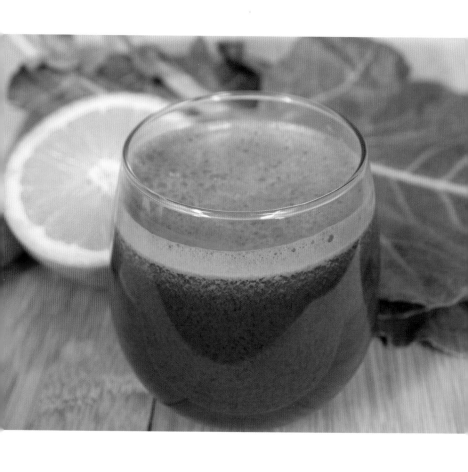

Southern Soul

Makes 1 glass

Just like mustard greens, collard greens help lower cholesterol and are an anticancer powerhouse. Strong-flavored leafy greens like these two examples are detoxifying, antioxidant, and anti-inflammatory, so include them in your diet (and your juices) as often as you can. You can learn to like them—if you don't already—by starting to consume them little by little.

1 cup collard greens
½ cup parsley
1 cup lettuce
½ cucumber
½ orange
1 carrot
2 celery ribs

   ◆ Process all the ingredients in a juicer and serve.

You may have noticed that most of our juices have a cucumber base. This veggie is mother nature's offering to juicers, as it has buckets of water and goes well with mostly anything. Chinese medicine uses it to dissipate heat, and as a diuretic, laxative, and detoxifying aid.

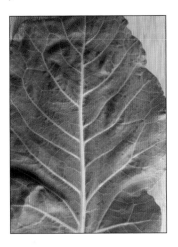

NOT SO GREEN, BUT SUPER HEALTHY

- Beet the Blues
- Beet-er Dandelion
- Save the Veggies
- Forever Young
- The Tummy Rub
- Cheers to Watercress
- Salad in a Glass
- Happy Belly
- Juice and Be Merry
- Yellow Submarine
- Healing Karma
- Not Your Regular OJ
- Hint of Mint
- Naturally Bright
- Cabbage Pear Kids
- A Walk in the Garden
- Belly Dancer
- Vitamin Cocktail
- Inner Guide
- Cleopatra's Night Tonic
- Glow like a Gem
- Monsoon Flower

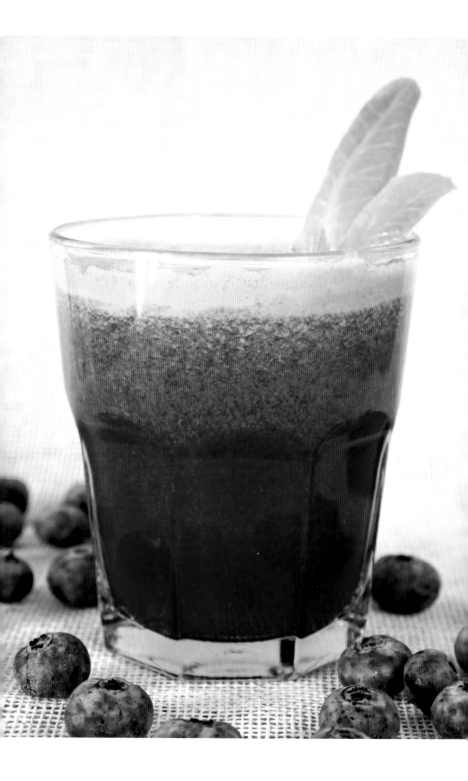

Beet the Blues

Makes 1 glass

If you're an eighties kid, the color of this juice may bring back memories of grape-flavored chewing gum rolls that came in hard plastic containers. Thankfully, in this case the cheerful color is not the result of scary chemicals and colorings, but of all the goodness stored inside blueberries and beets instead.

½–1 beet (with leaves, optional)
1 cup blueberries
½ heart of romaine
2 celery ribs
½–1 cucumber
½ apple
½-inch piece ginger, peeled

♦ Process all the ingredients in a juicer and serve.

When using beets, don't discard the greens. They are as good as the roots, and have a similar earthy flavor. In fact, beets were originally grown for their leaves, not their roots. You can use yellow or white beets, but nothing is more stunning than the intense magenta color that regular beets give to any juice.

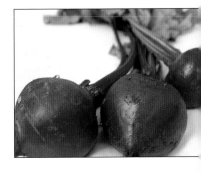

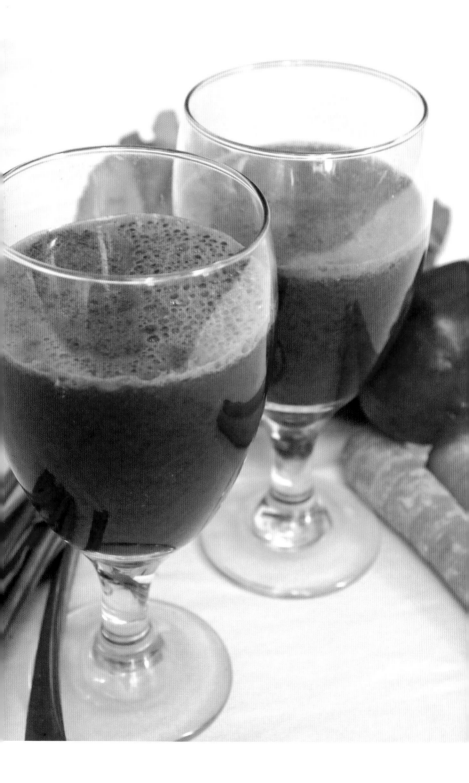

Beet-er Dandelion

Makes 1 glass

This intensely colored and flavored juice is not for the fainthearted. The bitterness of dandelion may put sweetness seekers off this drink, but for me, its superior detoxifying properties more than make up for it. No pain, no gain.

2 dandelion leaves
1 beet
1 carrot
½ cucumber
½–1 lemon
½ Granny Smith apple (optional)

♦ Juice all the ingredients and serve.

If you want the real hardcore version of this juice, have it without the apple. The beets and carrots already are rich in sugar, and more fruit only adds to it. However, if you really need it, you can add the fruit to get the benefits of the dandelion leaves past your taste buds.

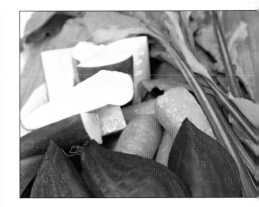

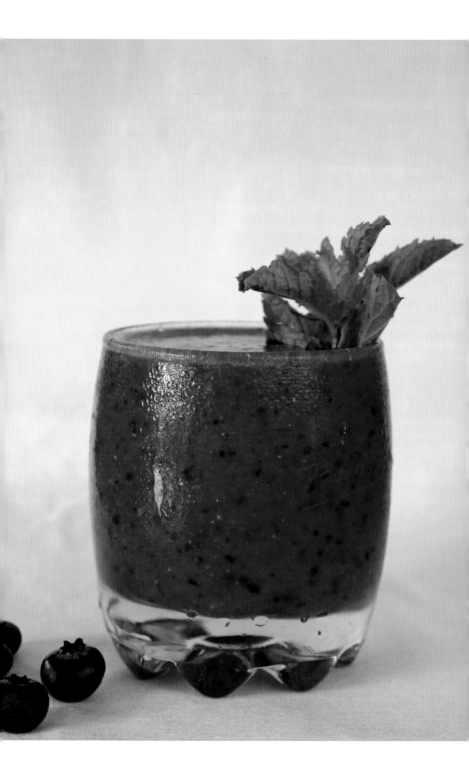

Save the Veggies

Makes 1 glass

This original juice was created by my Mom to recycle some leftover tomatoes and spinach that were being ignored in the fridge for a couple days. The sweetness added by the berries and pineapple water gave these veggies a 180-degree turn.

1 cup berries
1 tomato
1–2 cups spinach
½–1 cup pineapple water (page 55)

- ◆ Juice the first three ingredients.
- ◆ Mix with the pineapple water and serve.

Tomatoes are part of the nightshade group of foods, which have somewhat of a bad rep for having toxins that cause inflammation and pain. Defenders of nightshades, which also include potatoes, peppers, and eggplants, claim that the benefits far outweigh any potential problems caused by such low doses of these toxins. Our verdict? As long as you're not overdoing it, you can reap positive benefits from mostly anything.

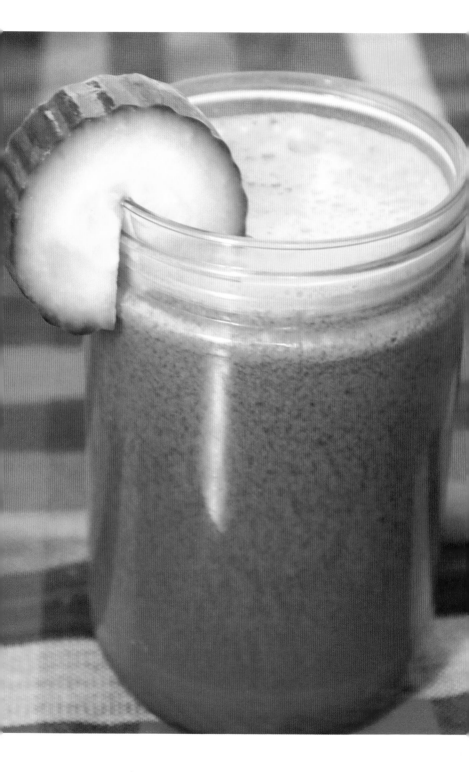

Forever Young

Makes 1 glass

The strong cilantro flavor in this refreshing juice is perfectly balanced by the sweetness of the carrots and the acidity of the lemon. The result is a truly enjoyable drink that will flush a huge amount of toxins out of your body. This is a recipe you may want to go back to again and again, not only for how much your liver loves it, but also for how much you do.

½ cucumber
1 large carrot
1 cup cilantro
Juice of ½ lemon

- ♦ Juice the cucumber, carrots, and cilantro.
- ♦ Squeeze the lemon into the juice and stir.

Who needs a cold beer when it's hot and muggy outside? The minerals in this juice will quench your thirst better than any other drink.

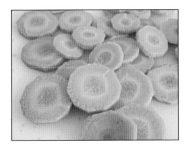

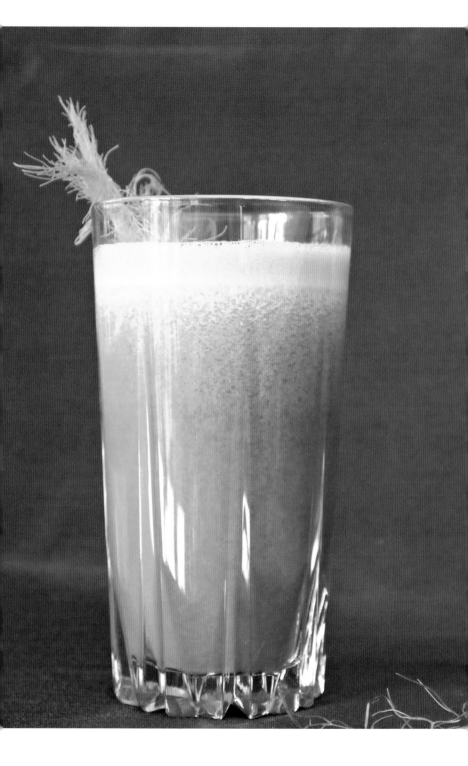

The Tummy Rub

Makes 1 glass

This green juice is an efficient cleanser and tonic of the hardworking yet delicate digestive system. Drink it half an hour before a heavy meal, as it stimulates your gut and gets it ready for action. You can also replace a meal with it if you're feeling heavy from a previous binge.

1 cup pineapple chunks
½ fennel bulb
½ cucumber
1 cup spinach
½ lemon

- Process all the ingredients in a juicer and serve.

Fennel has an aniseed flavor and, similar to that seed, aids digestion and prevents gas. It is also known to be a diuretic, reduce inflammation, and prevent cancer. As a food, only the round bulb is usually used, but for juicing use the bulb, stalks, and leaves. Everything goes.

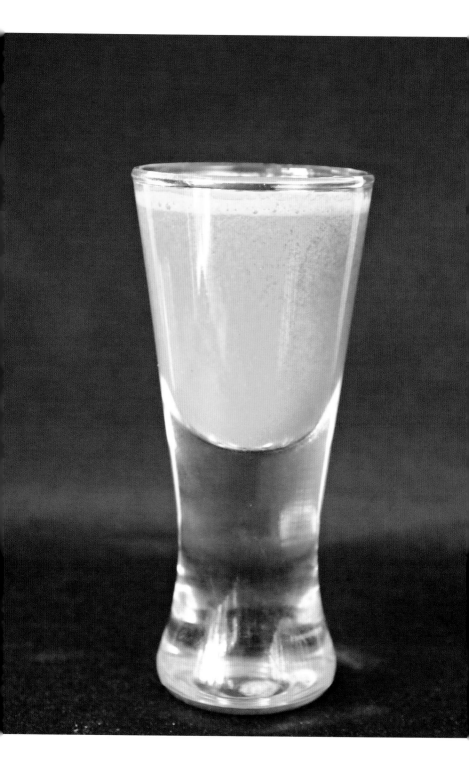

Cheers to Watercress

Makes 1 shot

The strong peppery taste of watercress has the spotlight in this juice, warming up your throat and stomach when you drink it. We rather enjoy it, although this may be too edgy for those who consider sweetness to be the only acceptable taste in a juice. Be brave and have it as a shot one day, or every day. If you like it, go ahead and have a whole glass (you may have to triple the recipe to get a decent-sized glass of it).

½ cup watercress
½ cup cucumber
½ cup carrot
¼ lime, peeled

◆ Juice all the ingredients and serve in a shot glass.

Watercress is an ace at detoxifying the liver and cleansing the blood. It is also a master antibiotic, improves eye health and night blindness, keeps your bones healthy, and prevents several kinds of cancer. Toast for health with this instead of booze, and you will be doing your liver a big favor.

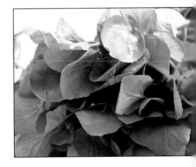

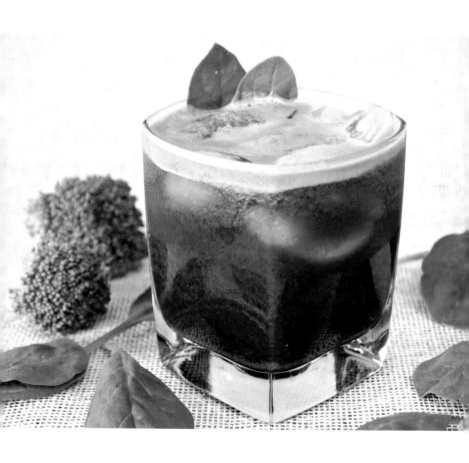

Salad in a Glass

Makes 1 glass

The color of this juice is as deep as the level of well-being it will bring to the new and improved you. Juice it once and your body will feel the difference. Juice it more often and you and everyone around you will notice its powerful effect.

1 cup broccoli
1 cup spinach
1 beet
1 apple
½ cucumber
½-inch piece ginger, peeled

◆ Process all the ingredients in a juicer and serve.

Boasting large amounts of sulfur, calcium, magnesium, iron, and vitamins, broccoli is a superb ingredient to include in juices and smoothies. Choose dark green heads and store them in the fridge inside a plastic bag to keep them from getting limp. Always try to use them before they start turning yellow.

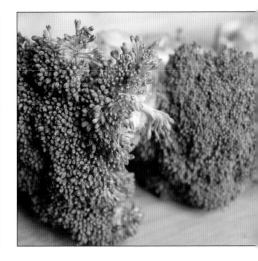

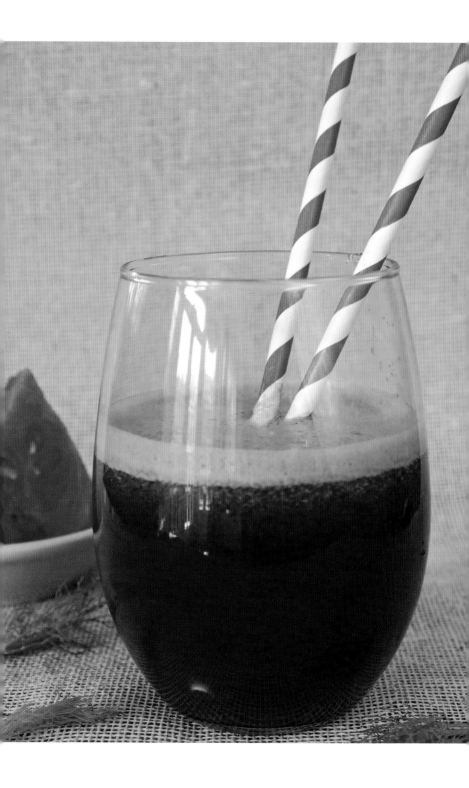

Happy Belly

Makes 1 glass

If you like an aromatic hint in your juice, this recipe is for you. Some people dislike the flavors of anise, licorice, fennel, and the like, but if they knew what wonderful digestive aids these are, maybe they would change their minds.

½ fennel bulb
1 cup watermelon, cubed and seeded
1 cup zucchini
1 cup spinach
1 cup parsley
½ lemon

- Process all the ingredients in a juicer and serve.

Like in tomatoes, the red color of watermelons are the result of their high lycopene content, which makes them especially important for the heart. My mom had a friend who had serious heart issues many years ago. She was put on a strict—and some thought crazy—watermelon diet. She lost forty pounds and healed her heart.

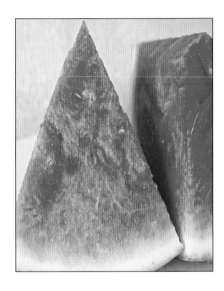

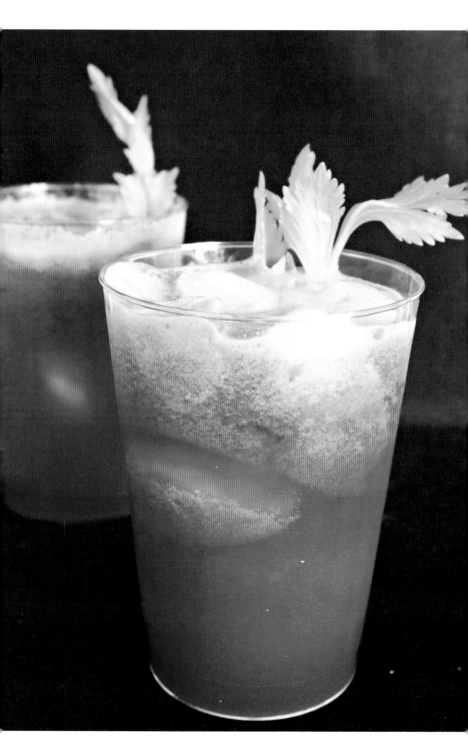

Juice and Be Merry

Makes 1 glass

Beets are one of the most detoxifying foods under the sun, as they are powerful cleansers of the bladder, kidneys, and liver. Anytime is good to have a tall glass of fresh beet juice, but take it one beet at a time as you build up your cleansing stamina.

1 beet
1 apple
2 celery ribs
½ cucumber
½–1 lemon

* Process all the ingredients in a juicer and serve.

Some cucumbers you buy at the grocery store may come covered in a thin layer of wax. You will have to take a close look to notice it, because it's transparent. When making juice, make sure you peel your cucumbers if they're not organic and if they have this waxy outer skin.

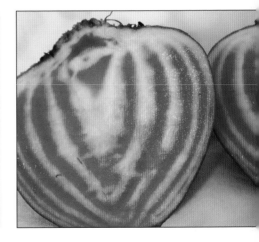

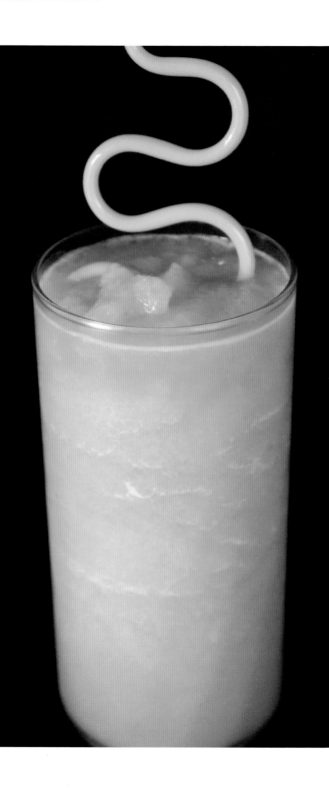

Yellow Submarine

Makes 1 glass

If you are having digestive issues and have tried everything without results, this may be your lucky day. Cabbage and pineapple work wonders for your body's oven, helping with uncomfortable issues like indigestion and heartburn. You won't even need to cover your nose to drink the sometimes intimidating cabbage juice, as the dominating sweetness of pineapple will come to the rescue.

2 cups cabbage
1 cup pineapple chunks
½ cucumber

* Process all the ingredients in a juicer and serve.

Despite its pale complexion, which makes it look not so interesting or potent, cabbage is very rich in sulfur, an antioxidant that is greatly detoxifying for the liver and increases the production of bile.

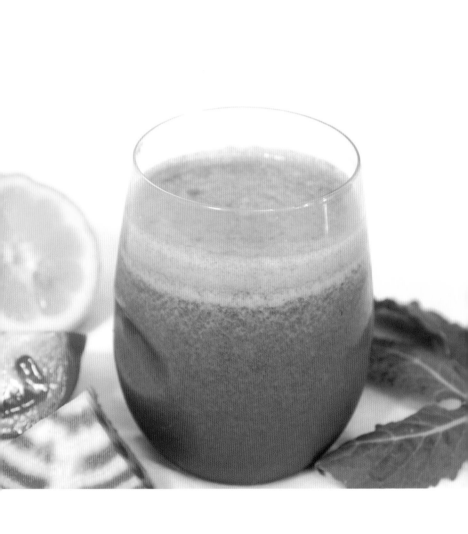

Healing Karma

Makes 1 glass

Depending on the type of beets you use, you will get a very different color when you make this juice. Beets are one of the most powerful liver tonics in the world. They power cleanse both the liver and the spleen, and help with more serious liver problems, such as cirrhosis.

2 tomatoes
1 beet
1 cup kale
½ heart of romaine
½–1 lemon

- ◆ Juice all the ingredients and serve.
- ◆ This juice is more enjoyable when cold, like a Bloody Mary, so add some ice cubes if you feel like it.

Rich in lycopene, tomatoes protect the liver and make it more efficient at metabolizing and removing toxins from the body.

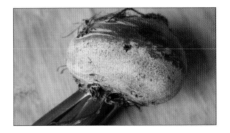

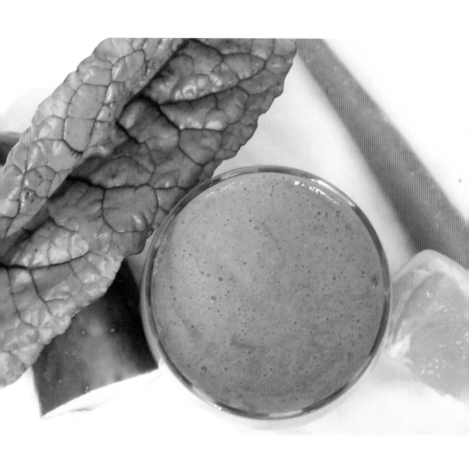

Not Your Regular OJ

Makes 1 glass

Our ancestors were wise when they got us in the habit of drinking a glass of freshly squeezed orange juice for breakfast, as this is one of the most effective ways to detoxify the body. Here, I've taken this nutrient-rich juice one step further by mixing it with cucumber, chard, and carrots. Drink it during the winter months, and you won't need tissues or cough drops ever again.

½ cucumber
4 chard leaves
1–2 carrots
1 orange, peeled

◆ Juice all the ingredients and serve.

Even though some root vegetables can be juiced with their leaves, some people believe that carrot leaves are toxic, and can cause symptoms such as elevated heart rate and blood pressure, among others. Better to err on the side of caution and avoid them.

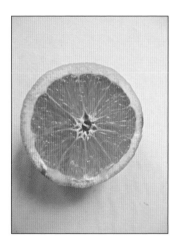

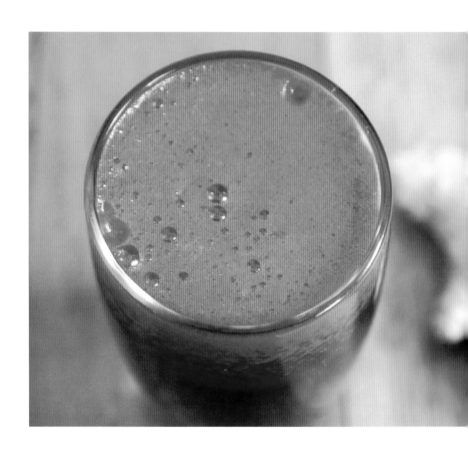

Hint of Mint

Makes 1 glass

The dominant flavors in this juice are those of the beet and the mint, and its potent detoxifying qualities come from all the ingredients used to make it, but particularly from those two. Beets and mint have blood-cleansing properties, and will literally refresh from the inside and out.

½ cucumber
½-inch piece ginger, peeled
½ apple
1 beet
1 sprig mint

- ◆ Juice all the ingredients and serve.

Ginger is one of the ingredients that we have a harder time finding in its organic version, so we usually peel it. This task is easier than you may think, and it doesn't even involve a knife. Simply push the skin down with the tip of a teaspoon, and it will easily come off.

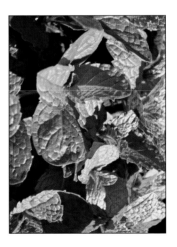

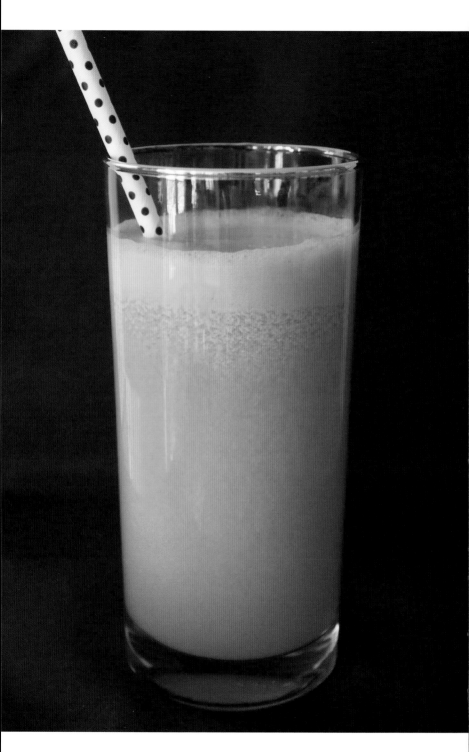

Naturally Bright

Makes 1 glass

I love drinking this vibrant juice simply because I find it delicious. The fact that carrots and grapefruits are such nutritional powerhouses doesn't hurt either. Depending on the kind of lettuce you use, the color will change from an opaque orange to a very bright one.

2 carrots
½ grapefruit, peeled
½ cucumber
2 cups escarole (or any other kind of lettuce)

◆ Process all the ingredients in a juicer and serve.

Do you remember when having half a grapefruit for breakfast every day was in vogue to lose weight? The reason for that trend was that this fruit is low in calories and sugar, and it also boosts the immune system with its high dose of vitamin C. To pick the juiciest grapefruit, try to find one that feels heavy for its size.

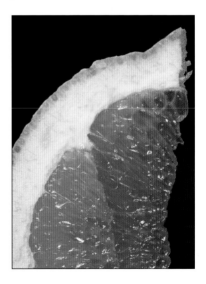

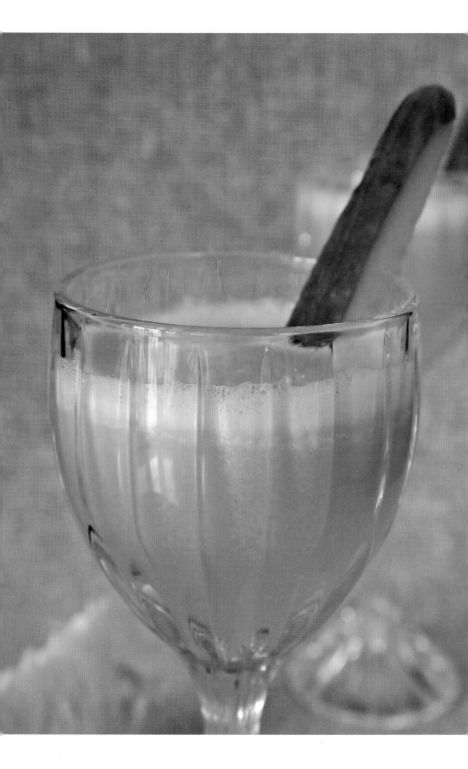

Cabbage Pear Kids

Makes 1 glass

Cabbage comes very handy when you cleanse, as it's a very affordable vegetable and may yield a good amount of juice depending on which one you pick. Give this juice a try and notice how good your stomach starts to feel, especially if you suffer from heartburn, gastritis, or peptic ulcers. In Chinese medicine, cabbage is used to treat constipation. The more of it you consume, the better.

2 cups cabbage
2 ripe pears
½ cucumber
½-inch piece ginger, peeled
½ lime, peeled

+ Process all the ingredients in a juicer and serve.

Want to look fresh and young? Ditch the Botox injections and get in the habit of juicing cabbage instead. This cruciferous vegetable helps in the production of collagen, the basis for younger-looking skin, and it also heals varicose veins.

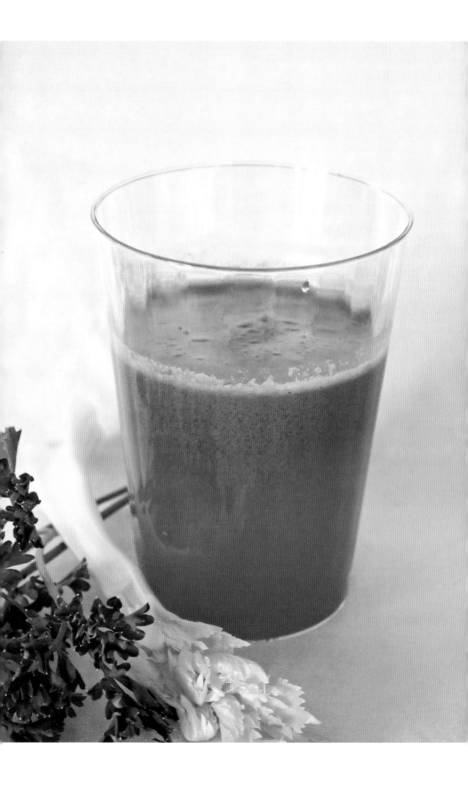

A Walk in the Garden

Makes 1 glass

My all-time favorite herb in the kitchen, the popular parsley, is rich in vitamins A, C, and K, protecting the kidneys and bladder. Its rejuvenating leaves have also been traditionally used to reduce high blood pressure. So stop using it as decoration only, and make it work for you by adding it to your juices.

3 carrots
4 celery ribs
2 cups parsley
½ cucumber

- Process all the ingredients in a juicer and serve.

Parsley and other herbs, such as cilantro, are so effective at detoxifying the body that you should start slowly when adding them to your juices. Be particularly careful—and even seek a doctor's advice—if you have kidney problems, as this herb will powerfully stimulate and cleanse them.

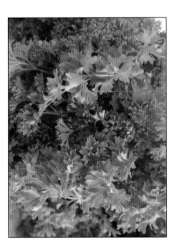

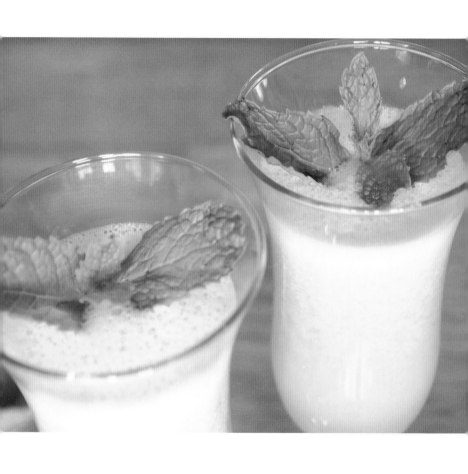

Belly Dancer

Makes 1 glass

Pineapple and mint should become your life partners if you have any digestive discomfort. Mint leaves are cooling and help relieve motion sickness, nausea, and cramps. Pineapple's bromelain (a potent digestive enzyme) is linked to a reduction in inflammation, rivaling commercial medications at this task.

1 cup pineapple chunks
2 sprigs mint
2 celery ribs
1 heart of romaine

- ♦ Process all the ingredients in a juicer and serve.

Pineapple is at its ripest point when very fragrant. Peel it and cut it in round slices or chunks. Keeping pineapple chunks in the freezer will make your life easier the next time you want to prepare a delicious juice or smoothie in the spur of the moment. Thaw it first if you're going to juice it.

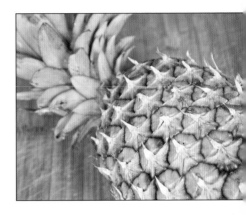

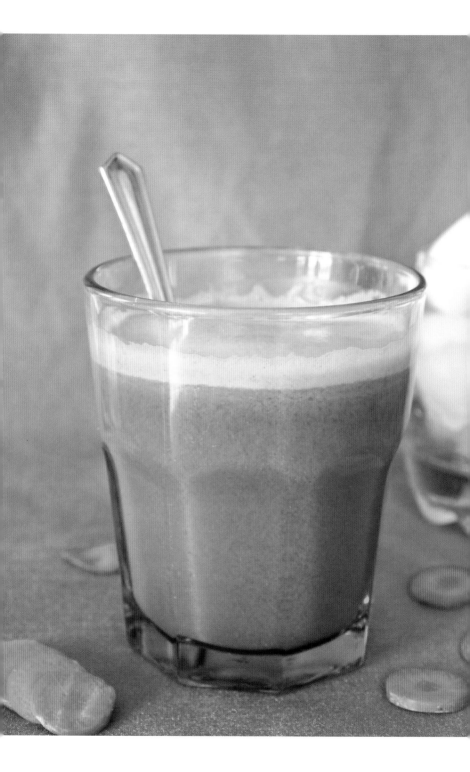

Vitamin Cocktail

Makes 1 glass

This antioxidant cocktail's key factor is the tartness of the grapefruit, which tempers the strong flavor of kale. Grapefruits are excellent for lowering cholesterol and don't have many calories, making them ideal for those watching their weight.

½ grapefruit, peeled
2 carrots
2 celery ribs
4 kale leaves
½-inch piece ginger, peeled

◆ Process all the ingredients in a juicer and serve.

The carotene in carrots is said to be best absorbed by the body if the carrots are cooked and mixed with a little oil. But for juicing, raw is obviously the way to go, and you will still get tons of benefits.

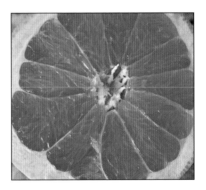

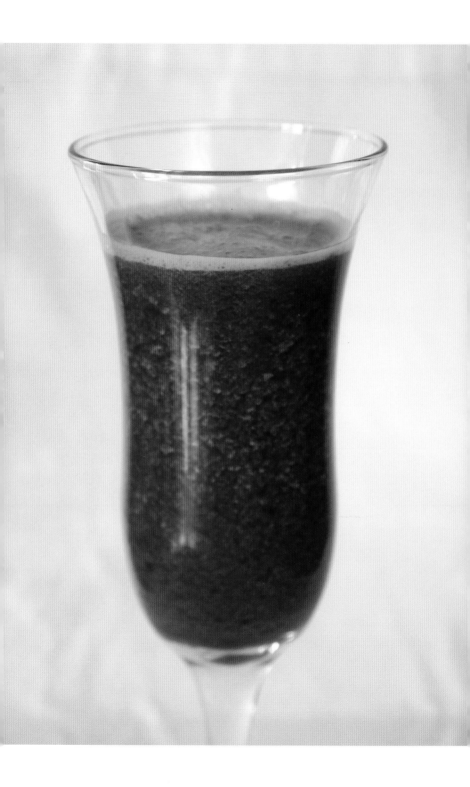

Inner Guide

Makes 1 glass

When you first start juicing, it's better to begin with a rookie-friendly recipe. Unless you have a very particular sense of taste, we can guarantee that you will enjoy this one, and that little by little you will start liking (and even craving) stronger ones. When that happens, it will be the moment to add spinach leaves or parsley, and then graduate to kale and wheatgrass.

2 cups blueberries
2 celery ribs
½ cucumber
½–1 lime

- ◆ Process all the ingredients in a juicer and serve.

Just as kale has the highest antioxidant content in the vegetable world, blueberries are the equivalent in the fruit world. A handful a day can protect you from many diseases, like high cholesterol, diabetes, cancer, heart disease, urinary tract infections, and memory loss. Keep them in the fridge or freeze them, and add them freely to salads, cereals, and smoothies.

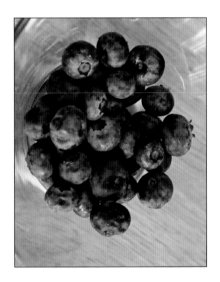

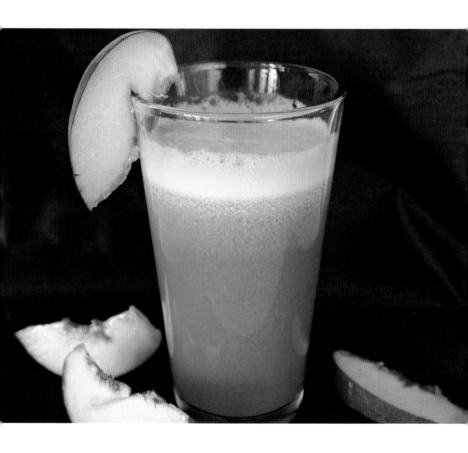

Cleopatra's Night Tonic

Makes 1 glass

Peach juice is creamy and sweet when the fruit is ripe. Its delicate fragrance is especially seductive in the summer, when they are in season. Combined with some relaxing lettuce, which makes you sleepy, this juice is best enjoyed in the evening, when you already have your jammies on. Teddy bear is optional.

3 ripe peaches
½ lettuce head
½ cucumber
½–1 lime

 ◆ Process all the ingredients in a juicer and serve.

Believe it or not, the humble lettuce has been around for thousands of years, and it was quite popular in ancient Egypt. Lettuce was highly appreciated for its relaxing powers, and some food historians say it was even used as a sleeping aid.

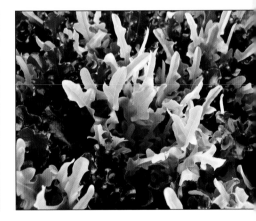

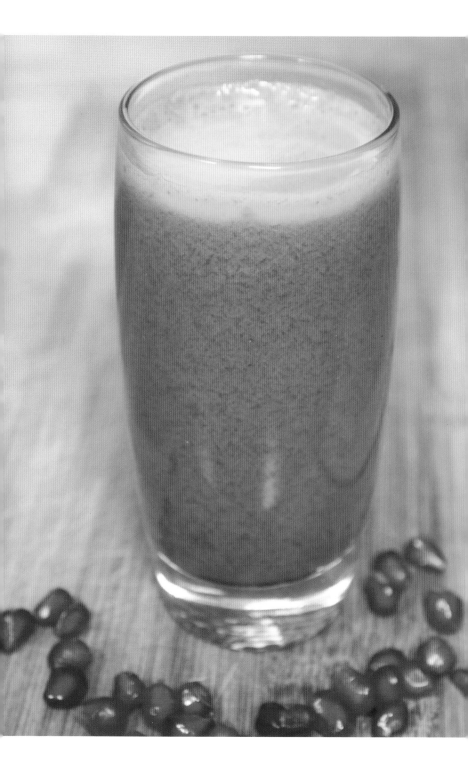

Glow like a Gem

Makes 1 glass

I have to admit I don't use pomegranate often enough in my recipes. But when I do, I love watching the way these sweet and tart seeds transform most juices. The magnetic color is telling of their great antioxidant properties. This explains why these precious seeds are one of the superfoods of our time.

2 cups pomegranate seeds
1 heart of romaine
2 carrots
½-inch piece ginger, peeled
½ lemon

- ◆ Juice all the ingredients and serve.

If you can't find fresh pomegranate, you may replace it with a good-quality, organic, sugar-free juice. Otherwise, replace it in this recipe with organic cherries or red grapes.

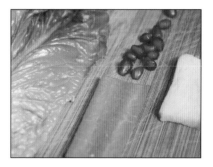

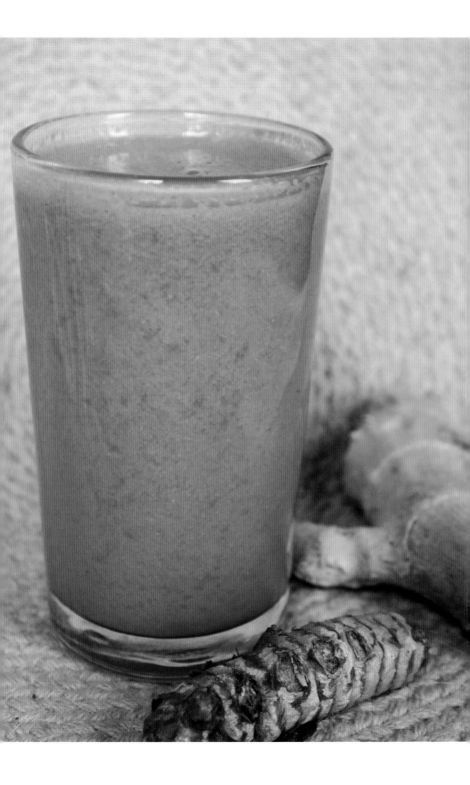

Monsoon Flower

Makes 1 glass

This juice was inspired by all the many vegetarian Indian dishes I've eaten throughout my life containing cauliflower and a vast array of spices. It is also the result of my newfound fascination with turmeric, Mother Earth's anti-inflammatory and antidepressant root. If you don't juice it, you can add it to your food, or make an infusion with it.

2 cups cauliflower
½ cucumber
1 orange, peeled
1-inch piece ginger, peeled
1-inch piece turmeric, peeled
2 carrots

+ Process all the ingredients in a juicer and serve.

Whenever you see fresh turmeric at the grocery store or the market, buy it! This intense yellow-orange spice is a real superfood, as effective at preventing and treating many ailments (such as arthritis) as the most sophisticated drugs. Turmeric is also a strong antioxidant, and may protect against Alzheimer's disease.

MORE SWEET AND FUN OPTIONS

- Sweetie Pie
- Strawberry Muse
- Bubbly Morning
- Honey Sol
- Kiwi Joy
- Chia Sweeper
- Summer Breeze
- Apple Crumble
- Tantalizing Lemongrass
- Sea of Greens
- Inca Life Force
- Apple Tart
- Peachy Keen

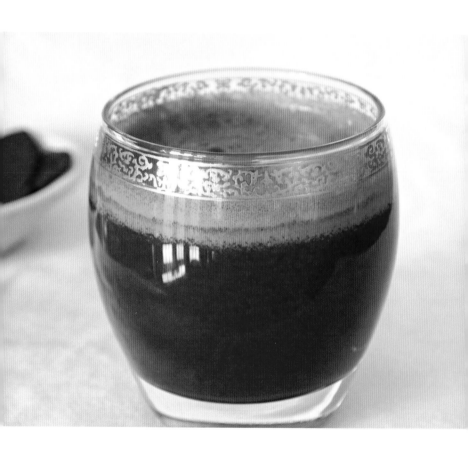

Sweetie Pie

Makes 1 glass

Are you surprised to find sweet potato in a juice recipe? The surprise should be that more people don't think about it! This vegetable's vibrant orange color shows what a great source of beta-carotene it is, making it a strong anticancer agent, and fabulous for healthy eyes, skin, and hair.

1 beet
½ grapefruit, peeled
½ cucumber
2-inch piece sweet potato
½-inch piece ginger, peeled

* Process all the ingredients in a juicer and serve.

Despite their name, the sweetness in sweet potatoes doesn't spike your sugar levels, making them ideal for diabetics. Who knew?

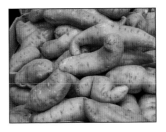

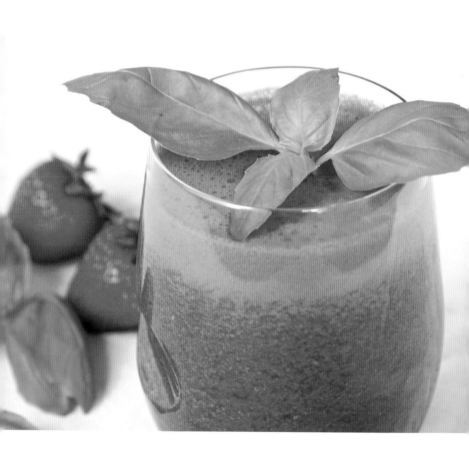

Strawberry Muse

Makes 1 glass

If you love the smell of basil when someone is making pesto in the kitchen, you will relish drinking its aromatic juice. This gorgeous drink will be a complete sensual experience, luring your senses of smell, sight, and taste alike.

½ cucumber
1 cup strawberries
1 beet
1 cup basil
1 teaspoon coconut oil (optional)

- Juice the cucumber, strawberries, beet, and basil.
- Add the coconut oil to the juice, stir with a spoon, and serve.

Basil has been appreciated in India and the Mediterranean for thousands of years for its digestive and antibacterial properties. These qualities make the pretty leaves a real treat for your body, which is able to rest and replenish more easily thanks to their help.

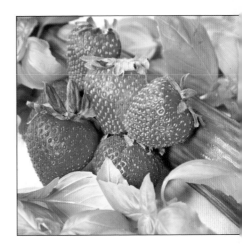

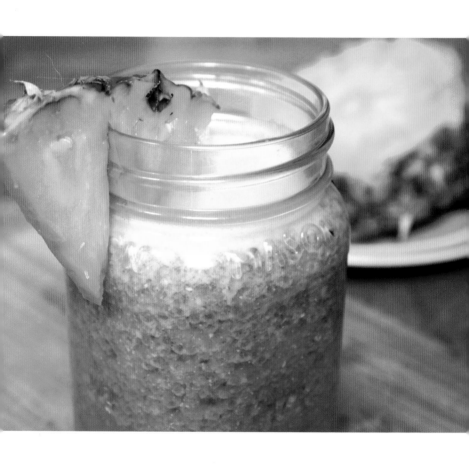

Bubbly Morning

Makes 1 glass

If you've never soaked chia seeds before, you're in for an exciting show. These tiny seeds absorb a lot of water, quickly plumping up with a jelly-like coating around each of them. These super bubbles will swipe out everything they stumble upon on their voyage through your gut.

1½ cups pineapple
2 celery ribs
1 cup kale
½–1 cup nut milk (page 41)
1 tablespoon chia seeds

- ◆ Juice the pineapple, celery, and kale.
- ◆ Mix the juice, nut milk, and chia seeds with a spoon.
- ◆ Let the chia seeds soak in this juice for 5 to 10 minutes, and serve.

This is a great juice to have first thing in the morning, as the fiber in the chia will get things moving and clean you out. The nut milk will keep you full and energized for several hours.

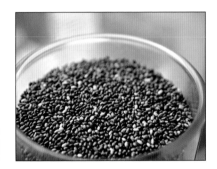

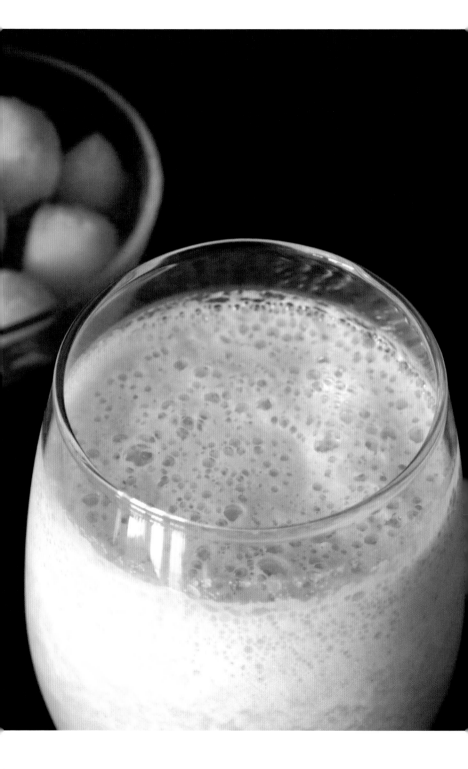

Honey Sol

Makes 1 glass

Honeydew melons are sweet as honey, just like their name implies. Including this yummy fruit in your juices and smoothies will lighten up and bring sweetness to even the sternest of them. By the way, I named this one after my dog. She has a honeydew effect on our lives.

2 cups honeydew, cubed
½ cucumber
½ heart of romaine
Juice of ½–1 lemon

- ◆ Process the honeydew, cucumber, and heart of romaine in a juicer.
- ◆ Add the lemon juice and serve.

Vary this juice easily by using an orange instead of the lemon. For a completely different flavor, substitute the lemon juice with a half teaspoon of ground cinnamon. And there you have it: three juices in one.

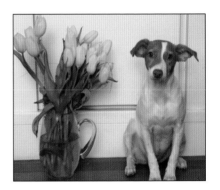

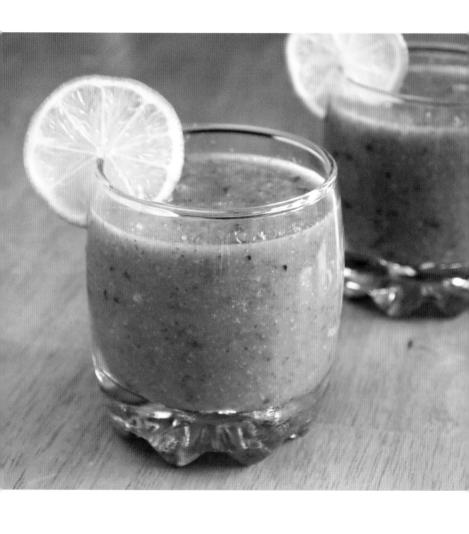

Kiwi Joy

Makes 1 glass

When it comes to juicing, you can find a solution for any problem you encounter. You don't like the flavor of a straight green juice? Add fruit to make it sweeter. The natural sugars of the fruit make you drowsy? No problem, add a nut milk that will help you stabilize your sugar levels. This is how this juice came about.

1 cup spinach
½ cucumber
1 kiwi, peeled
1 cup grapes
½ lemon
½ cup almond milk (page 41)

- Juice the first five ingredients.
- Stir in the almond milk and enjoy.

Once you get to know your fruits and veggies better, juicing them will be an easier task. For example, instead of peeling your kiwis, you will learn that cutting them in half and scooping the flesh out with the spoon is quicker. The same trick works with avocados.

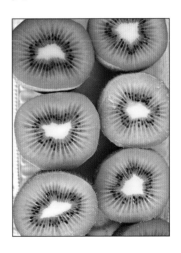

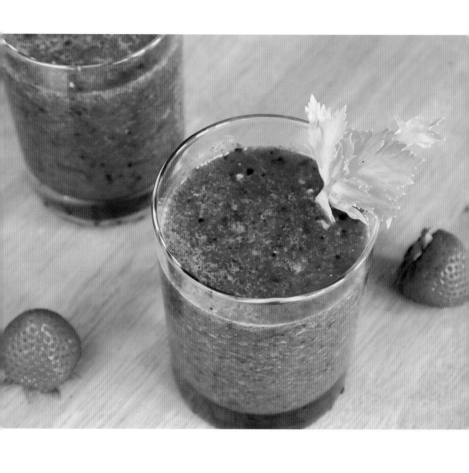

Chia Sweeper

Makes 1 glass

Homemade almond milk is a wonderful ingredient to have on hand when you want to make quick and healthy drinks that will keep you full throughout the day. Add chia to the mix, and you won't even remember the word "food" until your next meal.

1 cup watermelon, cubed and seeded
1 cup berries
2 celery ribs
½ lemon
½ cup almond milk (page 41)
1 tablespoon chia seeds

- Juice the first four ingredients.
- Add the almond milk and chia seeds, stir, and let the seeds soak for 5 to 10 minutes.

Would you ever have guessed that chia seeds are from the mint family? Surprise, surprise! Native to Guatemala and Mexico, these seeds were being munched on by the wise Aztecs long before the Spanish conquerors came to town in the sixteenth century. The high content of healthy oils in them probably gave them their name, which comes from the Nahuatl word *chian*, meaning "oily."

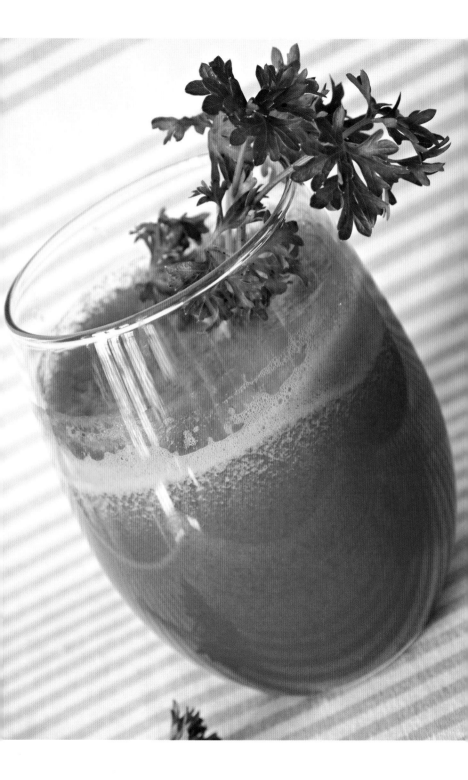

Summer Breeze

Makes 1 glass

Rich in chlorophyll, soothing to the digestive system, alkalizing, and a blood pressure regulator. These are just some of the qualities of this striking red juice. Not all juices will please every palate. This one, however, is most likely to be everyone's cup of tea.

2 cups watermelon, cubed and seeded
2 cups strawberries
1 cup parsley
1 lime

♦ Process all the ingredients in a juicer and serve.

When juicing parsley, it's better to start slowly. There's a big difference between adding a little chopped parsley on your bruschetta, and taking it in concentrated doses that go directly to your bloodstream. The juice of this innocent-looking herb is highly detoxifying, which may make you feel like you are having a bit of an out-of-body experience if it's the first time you are taking it in such high doses.

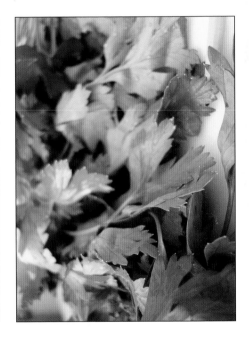

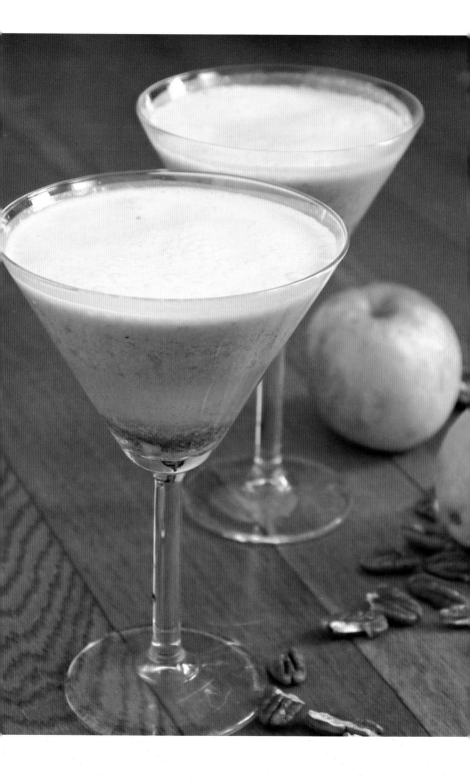

Apple Crumble

Makes 1 glass

Apples are known for cleansing the liver and gallbladder. Celery is a powerful diuretic. Ginger stimulates digestion, circulation, and sweating. Put these three healing ingredients together and you have a recipe made in detox heaven!

1 apple
2 celery ribs
1 cup escarole
½-inch piece ginger, peeled
½ cup nut milk (page 41) or seed milk (page 53)
1 tablespoon ground flaxseeds

- ◆ Juice the first four ingredients.
- ◆ Add the nut or seed milk and flaxseeds, and stir well with a spoon.

Boost the energetic power of this shake by adding hemp and maca powders to the blend. You can also add one teaspoon of chia seeds to each glass to literally swipe those toxins out of your body. Stir them in with a spoon and let the seeds sit for five to ten minutes, to give them enough time to absorb some water and grow.

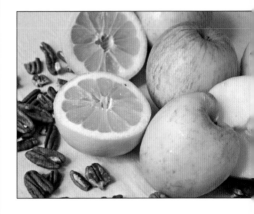

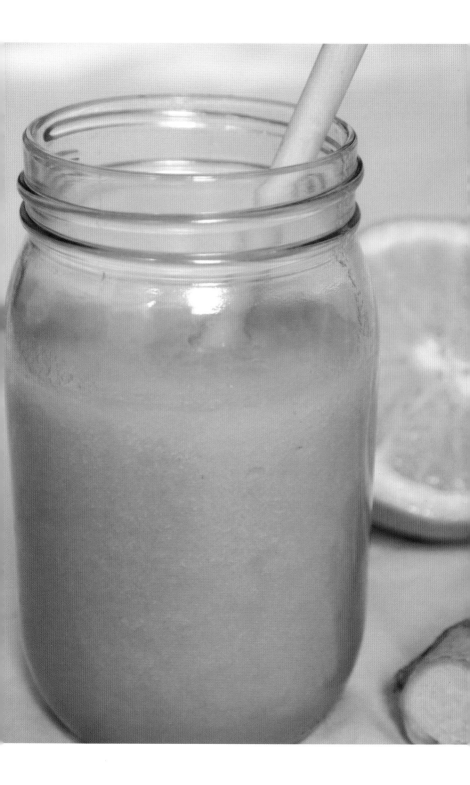

Tantalizing Lemongrass

Makes 1 glass

When I was a kid, I was once playing in our garden when I was suddenly struck by a hypnotizing lemon smell. We didn't have a lemon tree, and that's when I realized the culprit was a giant pot of vibrant lemongrass. Realizing this herb can be juiced has been as exciting a discovery as lemongrass was in the first place. It adds incredible depth to any juice, while also speeding up the detox process in the body.

½ cucumber
2 ripe peaches
1 orange, peeled
½-inch piece ginger root, peeled
1–2 lemongrass sticks

♦ Juice all the ingredients and serve.

You can add lemongrass to many of your juices. Sometimes you can even replace lemon with it. But smoothies are a different story. Ingesting the wood-like fiber of a lemongrass stick is not a pleasant experience.

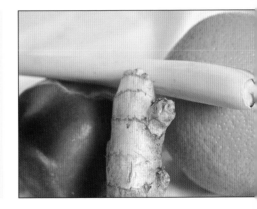

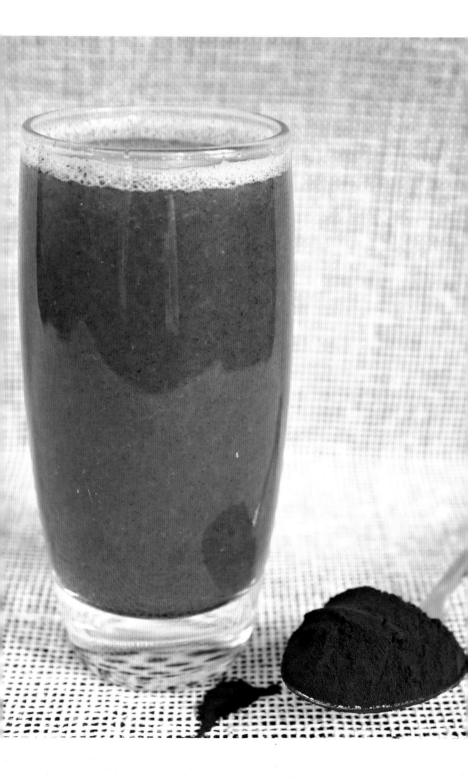

Sea of Greens

Makes 1 glass

Who needs to be artificially invigorated with energy drinks, when nature has given us all we need to feel our best? Coconut water is a miracle drink, said to resemble human blood plasma. Chlorella is a sea veggie that turns your pH alkaline, strengthens the body's natural defense mechanism, and detoxifies chemicals and heavy metals.

1 ripe mango
1 cup coconut water
1 teaspoon chlorella or spirulina (optional)

- ◆ Peel the mango, cut the pulp off the seed, and process it in a juicer.
- ◆ Mix the mango juice with the coconut water and the chlorella or spirulina.

You can use chlorella or spirulina interchangeably for this juice, or use them both, as you cannot overdose on these amazing microalgae. Just be mindful of the intense taste they will add to your juice.

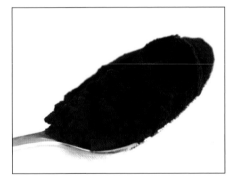

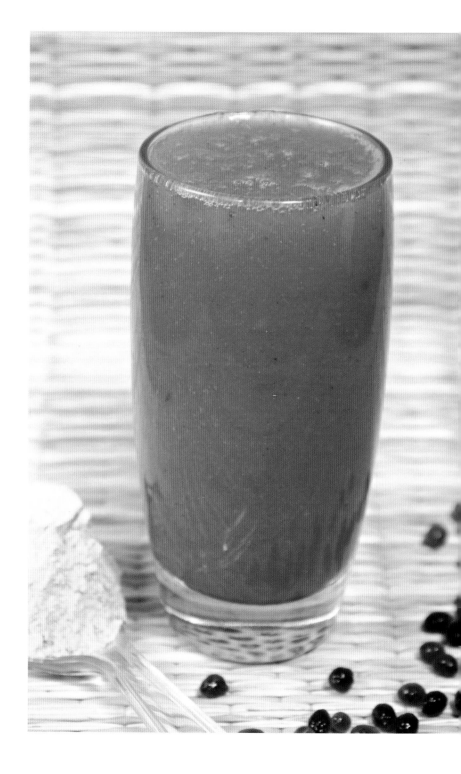

Inca Life Force

Makes 1 glass

This juice is a perfect way to start your day. The cleansing papaya will detoxify and nourish your cells, while also pacifying your digestive system. Add the radical energy of maca, and the diuretic pineapple water, and you'll be ready to go.

2–3 cups ripe papaya, peeled and cubed
1 cup pineapple water (page 55)
1 teaspoon maca powder (optional)

- Peel the papaya and process it in a juicer.
- Mix the juice, pineapple water, and maca, and serve.

Bring sexy time back to the bedroom by drinking maca on a daily basis. This strong sexual enhancer is known as "the Viagra of the Incas." If you have an embarrassing pimple too many or are chronically fatigued, maca could also help, as it provides out-of-this-world levels of energy, and regulates hormonal imbalances.

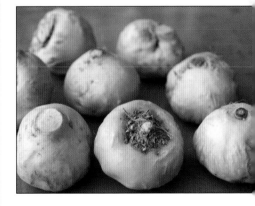

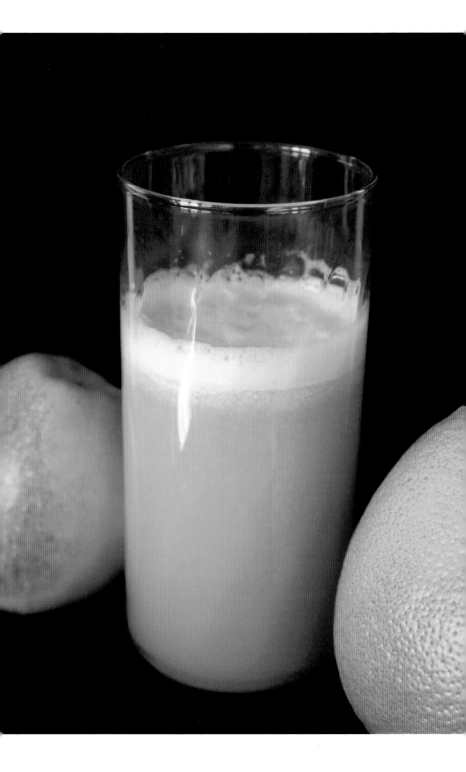

Apple Tart

Makes 1 glass

My family has always been a big fan of apple juice. My mom used to buy big pints of it all the time when I was a kid, and they would be gone in a matter of minutes. As much as we adore it, nothing compares to its freshly made version, especially when combined with a tart piece of grapefruit and the exotic heat of ginger.

1 apple
½ cucumber
3 celery ribs
½ grapefruit, peeled
½-inch piece ginger, peeled

- Process all the ingredients in a juicer and serve.

> When juicing citrus fruits, you can leave the skin on if you want because this is where a lot of the nutrients are found. The one exception is grapefruit, because the skin is far too bitter. Peel the fruit but try to keep the white pith that lies between the skin and the pulp. This way you will get most of this fruit's health in your juice.

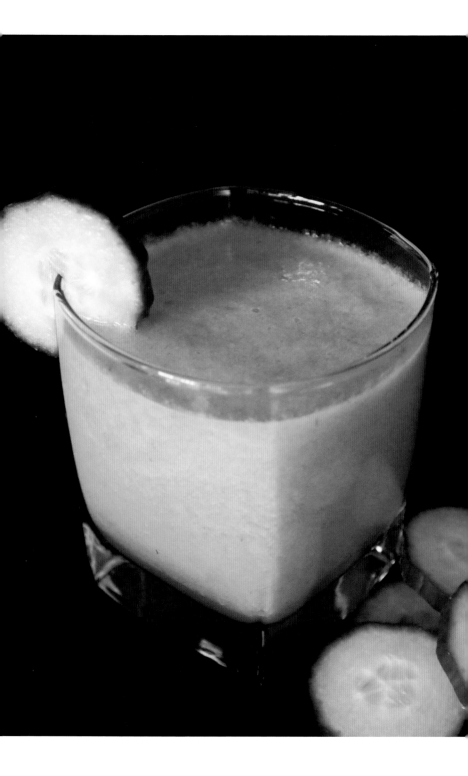

Peachy Keen

Makes 1 glass

It's easy to fall in love with the rich and creamy nectar that ripe peaches yield when juiced. Their velvety skin comes in different colors, and its softness is an indicator of the effect they have when consumed. You will literally get a peach-like complexion by juicing this top food for beautiful skin. So what are you waiting for?

3 ripe peaches
½ cucumber
3 celery ribs
1-inch piece ginger, peeled

◆ Process all the ingredients in a juicer and serve.

If peaches are underripe, they will be hard as stones and the juice they give won't be anything to write home about. Better to be patient and let them arrive at their sweet spot before using.

1 sprig mint

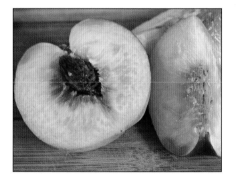

SMOOTHIES

- Dad's Fountain of Youth
- Avocado Delight
- Tea Time at Dawn
- Mother Earth's Dessert

- Grape Expectations
- Health Rocket
- God Save the Juice

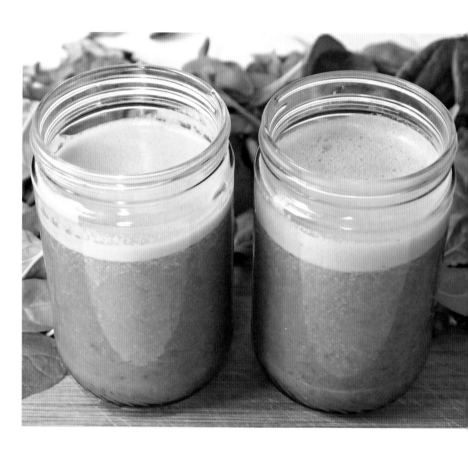

Dad's Fountain of Youth

Makes 1 glass

My seventy-nine-year-old father drinks this smoothie every morning as soon as he wakes up. For many years his breakfast consisted of a banana-and-milk smoothie. This was before I intervened and sent dairy into exile, replacing it with green juices, healthy fats, and fiber. Since he started drinking it this way, he has lost weight, he is healthier than he's ever been, his mood is more balanced, and even his voice is clearer. Nothing short of a miraculous fountain of youth.

2 celery ribs
1 cup spinach
4 lettuce leaves
½ cucumber
½ Granny Smith apple
½ banana
1 teaspoon flaxseeds (optional)
1 teaspoon chia seeds (optional)
1 teaspoon sesame seeds (optional)
1 teaspoon maca powder (optional)
1 teaspoon sacha inchi oil (optional)

- Juice the celery, spinach, lettuce, cucumber, and apple.
- Blend the green juice together with all the other ingredients.

If you suffer from depression or moodiness, you may want to experiment with maca. My mom's doctor once mentioned this powerful root's antidepressant qualities to her, but it wasn't until we saw the impressive improvements in my dad's mood after a few weeks of taking it religiously that we realized these claims were indeed true.

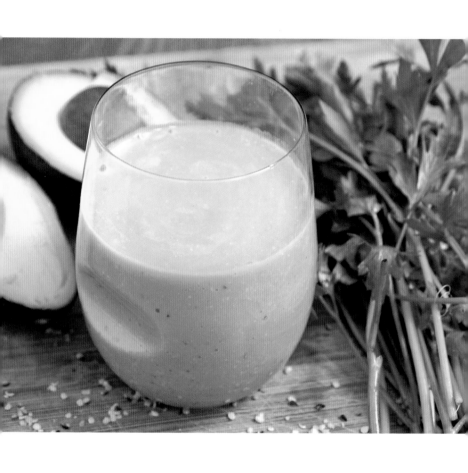

Avocado Delight

Makes 1 glass

Avocado is a fruit made in vegan heaven for all kinds of scrumptious dairy-free shakes. Its flavor goes almost unnoticed when mixed with other ingredients, and all it brings to the table is an appealing light green color and a creaminess that no milk or yogurt could compete with. Juicing newcomers: Don't be put off by the idea of adding avocado to your smoothies. Take the plunge and we promise it won't disappoint.

1 fennel bulb
1 kiwi, peeled
1 orange
1 cup parsley
½ avocado
1 tablespoon hempseeds or powder (optional)

♦ Juice the fennel, kiwi, orange, and parsley.
♦ Put this juice in a blender with the avocado and hempseeds. Process until smooth. If it's too thick, add water or the juice of ½ cucumber.
♦ Serve immediately. If you don't drink it soon the avocado will brown easily.

Choosing a good avocado is a simple endeavor. All you have to do is press it gently to see if your fingers sink into it slightly. If it's too soft (like butter), run away, as you will most likely find a blackened inside when you open it. If all you can find are hard-as-rock avocados, put them in a paper bag at room temperature until they soften.

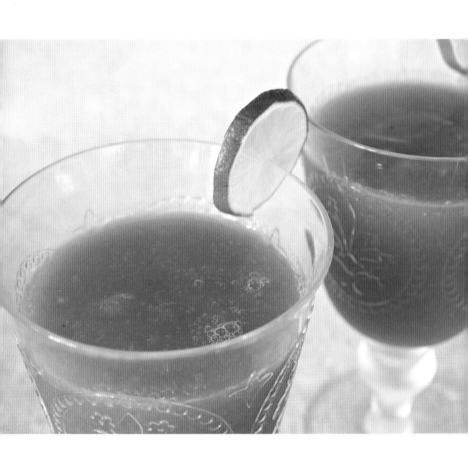

Tea Time at Dawn

Makes 1 glass

As I already mentioned, in Peru we like to drink fresh papaya and orange juice every morning for breakfast. In this case, we have added energetic green tea to the mix, as it speeds up the detox process in the liver cells while healing this important organ and burning fat. Green tea also helps wake you up, making it a great alternative to coffee.

1 cup papaya (with seeds), peeled and cubed
1 orange, peeled and cut in chunks
½–1 cup green tea, at room temperature

+ Process all the ingredients in a blender and serve.

Some people shy away from papaya because of its high sugar content, but they're missing out on the great health benefits this fruit offers, especially if you also add the seeds to your smoothies, which are highly detoxifying. To pick the best papaya, make sure it feels slightly soft to the touch.

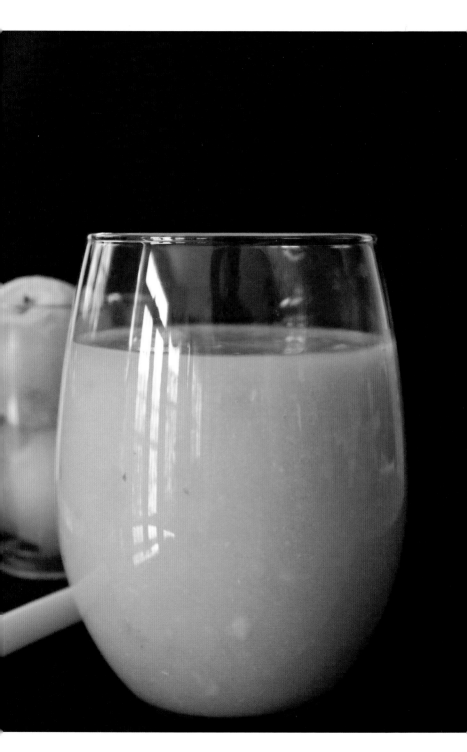

Mother Earth's Dessert

Makes 1 glass

Mangoes are nature's biggest gift for those of us who can't live without dessert, and you should keep one close if you know the day won't end without you falling into sinful, sugar-laden territories. If you ever feel like reaching for a slice of cake or cookie during a cleanse (or at any other time), have this instead. And if you're feeling extra naughty, replace the avocado with half a banana. We won't tell anyone.

½ ripe mango
1 ripe golden plum
1 cup coconut water
½ avocado

♦ Process all the ingredients in a blender until smooth, and serve.

Mangoes are used in the ancient Unani tradition to remove toxins from the body, treat anemia, and heal the nervous system. To achieve the desired rich color and taste in this smoothie, make sure you get a very ripe mango. Just look for one that is slightly soft when pressed, and very fragrant, even if it still looks green on the outside.

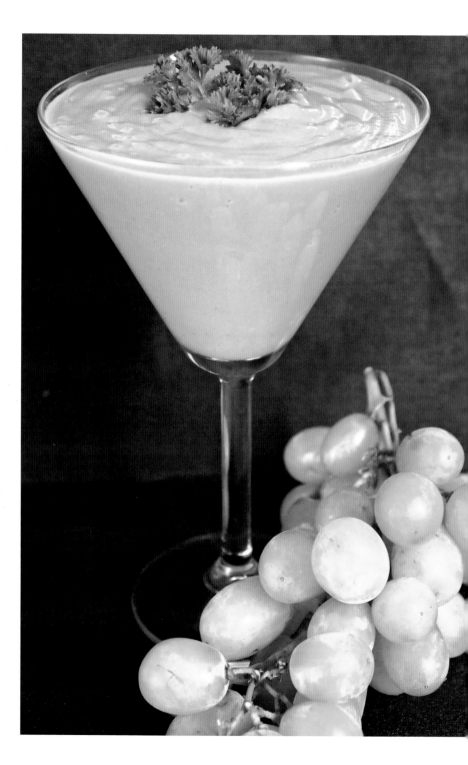

Grape Expectations

Makes 1 glass

Many women swear that their beauty secret is going on a grape mono-diet every now and then (this is a diet where you eat only grapes for several days). The Ayurvedic tradition also recommends fasting with only grape juice to reset the digestive fire and improve overall health.

2 cups green grapes
1 cup parsley
1 lemon
1 avocado

- Process the first three ingredients in a juicer.
- Blend this juice with the avocado.

Some of my friends think I'm crazy when I tell them that I make my juices creamy by adding avocado to them. I don't know what the big deal is, as this fruit is used in many dessert preparations and, most notably, to make ice cream. The truth is, you cannot judge it until you try it, and— trust me on this one—adding it to smoothies may very well be the best thing since sliced bread.

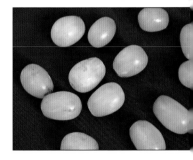

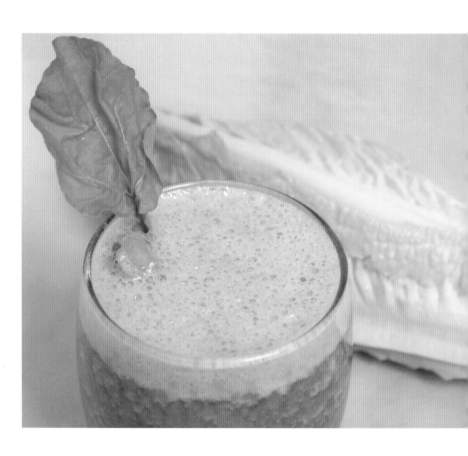

Health Rocket

Makes 1 glass

Also known as rocket or rucola, the bitter leaves of Arugula will shoot your health to the moon and back in one zesty drink. Arugula is one of my favorite greens, as it is nature's medicine packed into one pretty leaf. Do yourself a favor and include it in your juices and smoothies more often.

½ cucumber
2 cups arugula
1 heart of romaine
1 banana

- Juice the cucumber, arugula, and heart of romaine.
- Blend the banana and the juice together.

Arugula is packed with compounds that aid in detoxification, and it also has a cooling effect on the body. But that's not all. This sassy leaf has been used as a potent aphrodisiac for many centuries. Even the Greek philosophers and the Romans knew about the wonders of this love drug.

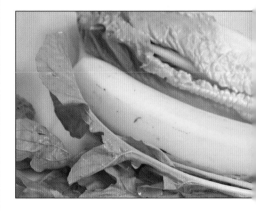

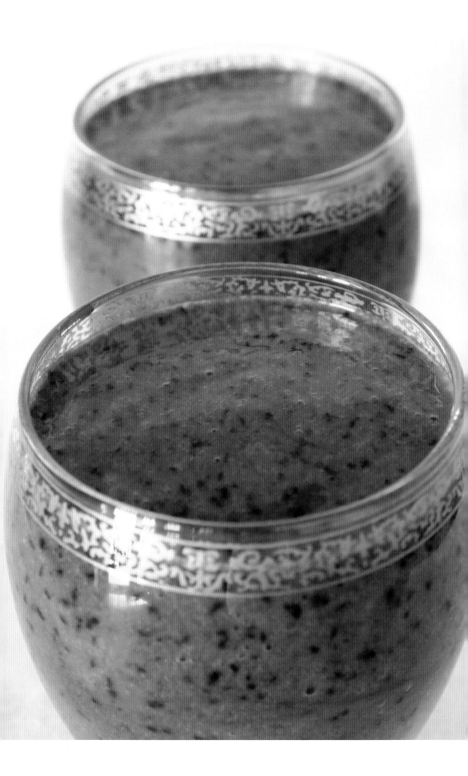

God Save the Juice

Makes 1 glass

The Brits got it right when they started drinking tea on a regular basis. They just picked the wrong kind! Regular tea certainly has many health benefits that make it worth the daily cup, but few things contain the antioxidant and detoxifying characteristics of green tea.

1 cup green tea
1 cup blueberries
1 cup kale
½ banana

- ◆ Prepare the green tea, and let it cool.
- ◆ Put all the ingredients in a blender and process until smooth, adding more green tea if needed.

Green tea also enhances the circulatory system and assists in weight loss by boosting your metabolism. During a body cleanse, feel free to have a cup between meals if you feel thirsty or hungry.

CHAPTER SEVEN:
DETOX PROGRAMS

A few guidelines to follow during a cleanse, and beyond:

- Start your day with a glass of Lemon-aid or Spice of Life.
- End your day with a glass of Hawaiian Elixir, or a cup of green or herbal tea.
- Between meals, drink as much water as you want, or drink green or herbal teas.
- Consult your doctor before starting any detox program.
- Whenever you don't see the name of a meal (breakfast, lunch, or dinner) in the daily plans, it means you should have a regular meal instead of a juice. Follow the guidelines in Chapter Four to know what to eat, and what to stay away from during a cleanse.
- If you can't find one of the ingredients for any of these juices, replace it with something else, or with a different juice.
- The juice snacks should be taken between meals.

THREE-DAY CLEANSES

Spring

- Day 1
    - Breakfast: Apple Tart
    - Snack: Simply Green
    - Snack: Green Up
    - Dinner: Save the Veggies
- Day 2
    - Breakfast: Apple Tart
    - Snack: Cheers to Watercress
- Snack: Simply Green
- Dinner: Save the Veggies

- Day 3
    - Breakfast: Apple Tart
    - Snack: Green Up
    - Snack: Cheers to Watercress
    - Dinner: Save the Veggies

Summer

- Day 1
  - Breakfast: Strawberry Muse
  - Snack: Simply Green
  - Snack: I Love Radishes
  - Dinner: Happy Belly

- Day 2
  - Breakfast: Strawberry Muse
  - Snack: Forever Young
  - Snack: Simply Green
  - Dinner: Happy Belly

- Day 3
  - Breakfast: Strawberry Muse
  - Snack: I Love Radishes
  - Snack: Forever Young
  - Dinner: Happy Belly

Fall

- Day 1
  - Breakfast: Grape Expectations
  - Snack: Green Is In
  - Snack: Simply Green
  - Dinner: Cabbage Pear Kids

- Day 2
  - Breakfast: Grape Expectations
  - Snack: Serious Business
  - Snack: Green Is In
  - Dinner: Cabbage Pear Kids

- Day 3
  - Breakfast: Grape Expectations
  - Snack: Simply Green
  - Snack: Serious Business
  - Dinner: Cabbage Pear Kids

Winter

- Day 1
  - Breakfast: God Save the Juice
  - Snack: Scarborough Fair
  - Snack: Simply Green
  - Dinner: Naturally Bright

- Day 2
  - Breakfast: God Save the Juice
  - Snack: Broccolini Genie
  - Snack: Scarborough Fair
  - Dinner: Naturally Bright

- Day 3
  - Breakfast: God Save the Juice
  - Snack: Simply Green
  - Snack: Broccolini Genie
  - Dinner: Naturally Bright

SEVEN-DAY CLEANSES

Spring

- Day 1
  - Breakfast: Avocado Delight
  - Snack: Simply Green
  - Snack: Green Up
  - Dinner: Thin like an Asparagus
- Day 2
  - Snack: Cheers to Watercress
  - Snack: Simply Green
  - Dinner: The Tummy Rub
- Day 3
  - Snack: Green Up
  - Snack: Cheers to Watercress
  - Dinner: The Tummy Rub
- Day 4
  - Breakfast: Avocado Delight
  - Snack: Simply Green

- Snack: Green Up
- Dinner: Thin like an Asparagus
- Day 5
  - Snack: Cheers to Watercress
  - Snack: Simply Green
  - Dinner: Salad in a Glass
- Day 6
  - Snack: Green Up
  - Snack: Cheers to Watercress
  - Dinner: Salad in a Glass
- Day 7
  - Breakfast: Avocado Delight
  - Snack: Simply Green
  - Snack: Green Up
  - Dinner: Thin like an Asparagus

Summer

- Day 1
  - Breakfast: Chia Sweeper
  - Snack: Simply Green
  - Snack: I Love Radishes
  - Dinner: Cool as a Cucumber
- Day 2
  - Snack: Forever Young
  - Snack: Simply Green
  - Dinner: Heart Chakra

- Day 3
  - Snack: I Love Radishes
  - Snack: Forever Young
  - Dinner: Heart Chakra
- Day 4
  - Breakfast: Chia Sweeper
  - Snack: Simply Green
  - Snack: I Love Radishes
  - Dinner: Cool as a Cucumber

- Day 5
  - Snack: Forever Young
  - Snack: Simply Green
  - Dinner: Healthy Mary
- Day 6
  - Snack: I Love Radishes
  - Snack: Forever Young

- Dinner: Healthy Mary
- Day 7
  - Breakfast: Chia Sweeper
  - Snack: Simply Green
  - Snack: I Love Radishes
  - Dinner: Cool as a Cucumber

Fall

- Day 1
  - Breakfast: Health Rocket
  - Snack: Green Is In
  - Snack: Simply Green
  - Dinner: Berry Good
- Day 2
  - Snack: Serious Business
  - Snack: Green Is In
  - Dinner: Holy Kale
- Day 3
  - Snack: Simply Green
  - Snack: Serious Business
  - Dinner: Holy Kale
- Day 4
  - Breakfast: Health Rocket
  - Snack: Green Is In

- Snack: Simply Green
- Dinner: Berry Good
- Day 5
  - Snack: Serious Business
  - Snack: Green Is In
  - Dinner: Hint of Mint
- Day 6
  - Snack: Simply Green
  - Snack: Serious Business
  - Dinner: Hint of Mint
- Day 7
  - Breakfast: Health Rocket
  - Snack: Green Is In
  - Snack: Simply Green
  - Dinner: Berry Good

Winter

- Day 1
  - Breakfast: Bubbly Morning
  - Snack: Scarborough Fair
  - Snack: Simply Green
  - Dinner: Vitamin Cocktail

- Day 2
  - Snack: Broccolini Genie
  - Snack: Scarborough Fair
  - Dinner: Southern Soul

- Day 3
    - Snack: Simply Green
    - Snack: Broccolini Genie
    - Dinner: Southern Soul
- Day 4
    - Breakfast: Bubbly Morning
    - Snack: Scarborough Fair
    - Snack: Simply Green
    - Dinner: Vitamin Cocktail
- Day 5
    - Snack: Broccolini Genie
    - Snack: Scarborough Fair
- Dinner: Apple Crumble
- Day 6
    - Snack: Simply Green
    - Snack: Broccolini Genie
    - Dinner: Apple Crumble
- Day 7
    - Breakfast: Bubbly Morning
    - Snack: Scarborough Fair
    - Snack: Simply Green
    - Dinner: Vitamin Cocktail

FOURTEEN-DAY CLEANSES

Spring

- Day 1
    - Breakfast: Belly Dancer
    - Snack: Simply Green
    - Snack: Green Up
    - Dinner: Not Your Regular OJ
- Day 2
    - Snack: Simply Green
    - Snack: Cheers to Watercress
    - Dinner: A Walk in the Garden
- Day 3
    - Snack: Simply Green
    - Snack: Twist and Sprout
- Day 4
    - Snack: Simply Green
    - Snack: Green Up
    - Dinner: Yellow Submarine
- Day 5
    - Breakfast: Belly Dancer
    - Snack: Simply Green
    - Snack: Cheers to Watercress
    - Dinner: Not Your Regular OJ
- Day 6
    - Snack: Simply Green
    - Snack: Twist and Sprout
    - Dinner: A Walk in the Garden

- Day 7
  - Snack: Simply Green
  - Snack: Green Up

- Day 8
  - Snack: Simply Green
  - Snack: Cheers to Watercress
  - Dinner: Yellow Submarine

- Day 9
  - Breakfast: Belly Dancer
  - Snack: Simply Green
  - Snack: Twist and Sprout
  - Dinner: Not Your Regular OJ

- Day 10
  - Snack: Simply Green
  - Snack: Green Up
  - Dinner: A Walk in the Garden

- Day 11
  - Snack: Simply Green
  - Snack: Cheers to Watercress

- Day 12
  - Snack: Simply Green
  - Snack: Twist and Sprout
  - Dinner: Yellow Submarine

- Day 13
  - Breakfast: Belly Dancer
  - Snack: Simply Green
  - Snack: Green Up
  - Dinner: Not Your Regular OJ

- Day 14
  - Snack: Simply Green
  - Snack: Cheers to Watercress
  - Dinner: A Walk in the Garden

Summer

- Day 1
  - Breakfast: Beet the Blues
  - Snack: Simply Green
  - Snack: Forever Young
  - Dinner: Beet-er Dandelion

- Day 2
  - Snack: Simply Green
  - Snack: I Love Radishes
  - Dinner: Cleopatra's Night Tonic

- Day 3
  - Snack: Simply Green
  - Snack: Sweetchini

- Day 4
  - Snack: Simply Green
  - Snack: Forever Young
  - Dinner: Healing Karma

- Day 5
  - Breakfast: Beet the Blues
  - Snack: Simply Green
  - Snack: I Love Radishes
  - Dinner: Beet-er Dandelion

- Day 6
  - Snack: Simply Green
  - Snack: Sweetchini
  - Dinner: Cleopatra's Night Tonic

- Day 7
  - Snack: Simply Green
  - Snack: Forever Young

- Day 8
  - Snack: Simply Green
  - Snack: I Love Radishes
  - Dinner: Healing Karma

- Day 9
  - Breakfast: Beet the Blues
  - Snack: Simply Green
  - Snack: Sweetchini
  - Dinner: Beet-er Dandelion

- Day 10
  - Snack: Simply Green
  - Snack: Forever Young
  - Dinner: Cleopatra's Night Tonic

- Day 11
  - Snack: Simply Green
  - Snack: I Love Radishes

- Day 12
  - Snack: Simply Green
  - Snack: Sweetchini
  - Dinner: Healing Karma

- Day 13
  - Breakfast: Beet the Blues
  - Snack: Simply Green
  - Snack: Forever Young
  - Dinner: Beet-er Dandelion

- Day 14
  - Snack: Simply Green
  - Snack: I Love Radishes
  - Dinner: Cleopatra's Night Tonic

Fall

- Day 1
  - Breakfast: Dad's Fountain of Youth
  - Snack: Simply Green
  - Snack: Green Is In
  - Dinner: Better than a V8

- Day 2
  - Snack: Simply Green
  - Snack: Serious Business
  - Dinner: Glow like a Gem

- Day 3
  - Snack: Simply Green
  - Snack: Pear-fect Health

- Day 4
  - Snack: Simply Green
  - Snack: Green Is In
  - Dinner: The Sweet Smell of Success

- Day 5
  - Breakfast: Dad's Fountain of Youth
  - Snack: Simply Green
  - Snack: Serious Business
  - Dinner: Better than a V8

- Day 6
  - Snack: Simply Green
  - Snack: Pear-fect Health
  - Dinner: Glow like a Gem

- Day 7
  - Snack: Simply Green
  - Snack: Green Is In

- Day 8
  - Snack: Simply Green
  - Snack: Serious Business
  - Dinner: The Sweet Smell of Success

- Day 9
  - Breakfast: Dad's Fountain of Youth
  - Snack: Simply Green
  - Snack: Pear-fect Health
  - Dinner: Better than a V8

- Day 10
  - Snack: Simply Green
  - Snack: Green Is In
  - Dinner: Glow like a Gem

- Day 11
  - Snack: Simply Green
  - Snack: Serious Business

- Day 12
  - Snack: Simply Green
  - Snack: Pear-fect Health
  - Dinner: The Sweet Smell of Success

- Day 13
  - Breakfast: Dad's Fountain of Youth
  - Snack: Simply Green
  - Snack: Green Is In
  - Dinner: Better than a V8

- Day 14
  - Snack: Simply Green
  - Snack: Serious Business
  - Dinner: Glow like a Gem

Winter

- Day 1
  - Breakfast: Green Raw-volution
  - Snack: Simply Green
  - Snack: Broccolini Genie
  - Dinner: Sweetie Pie

- Day 2
  - Snack: Simply Green
  - Snack: Scarborough Fair
  - Dinner: Juice and Be Merry

- Day 3
  - Snack: Simply Green
  - Snack: All You Need Is Kale

- Day 4
  - Snack: Simply Green
  - Snack: Broccolini Genie
  - Dinner: Apple Crumble

- Day 5
  - Breakfast: Green Raw-volution
  - Snack: Simply Green
  - Snack: Scarborough Fair
  - Dinner: Sweetie Pie

- Day 6
  - Snack: Simply Green
  - Snack: All You Need Is Kale
  - Dinner: Juice and Be Merry
- Day 7
  - Snack: Simply Green
  - Snack: Broccolini Genie
- Day 8
  - Snack: Simply Green
  - Snack: Scarborough Fair
  - Dinner: Apple Crumble
- Day 9
  - Breakfast: Green Raw-volution
  - Snack: Simply Green
  - Snack: All You Need Is Kale
  - Dinner: Sweetie Pie
- Day 10
  - Snack: Simply Green
  - Snack: Broccolini Genie
  - Dinner: Juice and Be Merry
- Day 11
  - Snack: Simply Green
  - Snack: Scarborough Fair
- Day 12
  - Snack: Simply Green
  - Snack: All You Need Is Kale
  - Dinner: Apple Crumble
- Day 13
  - Breakfast: Green Raw-volution
  - Snack: Simply Green
  - Snack: Broccolini Genie
  - Dinner: Sweetie Pie
- Day 14
  - Snack: Simply Green
  - Snack: Scarborough Fair
  - Dinner: Core Balance

RESOURCES

BOOKS

- *100 Best Health Foods*, LOVE FOOD 2009
- *La Almendra y Otros Frutos Secos* by Maria Luengo, Editorial Oceano 2009
- *Ayurveda* by Robert Svoboda, Editorial Kairos 1994
- *The Big Book of Juices* by Natalie Savona, Duncan Baird 2010
- *The China Study* by T. Colin Campbell and Thomas M. Campbell II, BenBella Books 2006
- *Crazy Sexy Diet* by Kris Carr, Skirt! 2011
- *Crazy Sexy Kitchen* by Kris Carr with Chad Sarno, Hay House 2012
- *The FastDiet* by Michael Mosley and Mimi Spencer, Atria Books 2013
- *The Healthy Green Drink Diet* by Jason Manheim, Skyhorse Publishing 2012
- *In Defense of Food* by Michael Pollan, Penguin Books 2009
- *The Liver Cleansing Diet* by Sandra Cabot, SCB International 2008
- *Perfect Health* by Deepak Chopra, Three Rivers Press 2000
- *Peruvian Power Foods* by Manuel Villacorta, MS, RD, and Jamie Shaw, Health Communications Inc. 2013
- *Raw Energy* by Stephanie Tourles, Storey Publishing 2009
- *Secrets of Longevity* by Maoshing Ni, Chronicle Books 2006
- *The Whole Truth Eating and Recipe Guide* by Andrea Beaman, 2006

ONLINE RESOURCES

- www.forksoverknives.com
- www.psychologyofeating.com
- www.kriscarr.com
- www.thehealthyapple.com
- www.prevention.com
- www.life.gaiam.com
- www.undergroundhealth.com
- www.eatlifewhole.com
- www.thedetoxdiva.com
- www.naturalnews.com
- www.blog.jaykordich.com
- www.foodmatters.tv
- www.doctoroz.com
- www.whfoods.com
- www.yogahealer.com

RECIPE INDEX

A Walk in the Garden, 127
All You Need Is Kale, 73
Apple Crumble, 157
Apple Tart, 165
Avocado Delight, 173

Beet the Blues, 97
Beet-er Dandelion, 99
Belly Dancer, 129
Berry Good, 87
Better than a V8, 79
Broccolini Genie, 71
Bubbly Morning, 147

Cabbage Pear Kids, 125
Cheers to Watercress, 107
Chia Sweeper, 153
Cleopatra's Night Tonic, 135
Cool as a Cucumber, 53

Dad's Fountain of Youth, 171

Forever Young, 103

Glow like a Gem, 137
God Save the Juice, 183
Grape Expectations, 179
Green Is In, 55
Green Raw-volution, 67
Green Up, 63

Happy Belly, 111

Hawaiian Elixir (a.k.a. Pineapple Water), 49
Healing Karma, 117
Health Nut (a.k.a. Nut Milk), 41
Health Rocket, 181
Healthy Mary, 65
Heart Chakra, 91
Hint of Mint, 121
Holy Kale, 57
Honey Sol, 149

I Love Radishes, 77
Inca Life Force, 163
Inner Guide, 133

Juice and Be Merry, 113

Kiwi Joy, 151

Lemon-aid, 43

Monsoon Flower, 139
Mother Earth's Dessert, 177

Naturally Bright, 123
Not Your Regular OJ, 119

Peachy Keen, 167
Pear-fect Health, 85

Salad in a Glass, 109
Save the Veggies, 101
Scarborough Fair, 81

Sea of Greens, 161

Serious Business, 89

Simply Green, 59

Southern Soul, 93

Spice of Life, 45

Strawberry Muse, 145

Summer Breeze, 155

Super Seed Me (a.k.a. Seed Milk), 47

Sweet Smell of Success, The, 83

Sweetchini, 61

Sweetie Pie, 143

Tantalizing Lemongrass, 159

Tea Time at Dawn, 175

Thin like an Asparagus, 69

Tummy Rub, The, 105

Twist and Sprout, 75

Vitamin Cocktail, 131

Yellow Submarine, 115